791.07

AQA AS

Physical Education

Carl Atherton   Symond Burrows   Sue Young

Philip Allan Updates, an imprint of Hodder Education, part of Hachette Livre UK, Market Place, Deddington, Oxfordshire OX15 0SE

Orders

Bookpoint Ltd, 130 Milton Park, Abingdon, Oxfordshire OX14 4SB
tel: 01235 827720
fax: 01235 400454
e-mail: uk.orders@bookpoint.co.uk

Lines are open 9.00 a.m.–5.00 p.m., Monday to Saturday, with a 24-hour message answering service. You can also order through the Philip Allan Updates website: www.philipallan.co.uk

© Philip Allan Updates 2008

ISBN 978-1-84489-643-1

Impression number   5 4 3 2 1
Year   2012 2011 2010 2009 2008

Printed in Italy.

Hachette Livre UK's policy is to use papers that are natural, renewable and recyclable products and made from wood grown in sustainable forests. The logging and manufacturing processes are expected to conform to the environmental regulations of the country of origin.

P01150

Contents

Chapter 9 Theories of learning

Opportunities for participation

Chapter 10 Characteristics and objectives of physical activity

Chapter 11 Facility provision

Chapter 12 Increasing participation

Chapter 13 Barriers to participation

Unit 2 Analysis and evaluation of physical activity as a performer and/or in adopted roles

Answers

Index

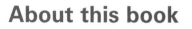

Introduction

About this book

This textbook is written for students following the AQA AS specification in PE.

The topics, which appear in the same order as in the specification, are explained clearly. Links to practical examples will help you to relate this theory to your own sporting experiences.

Each chapter contains a number of features designed to aid your understanding of the requirements of the AQA AS PE course.

- **Aims and objectives.** Each chapter begins with a clear outline of the subject matter and main topics covered.
- **Key terms.** Concise definitions of important terms are given throughout the book. A clear understanding of the key terms will reduce your chances of producing irrelevant answers in your exam, and hopefully earn more marks.
- **Top tips.** The authors use their considerable experience as teachers and examiners to provide useful pointers to help your exam performance and to avoid potential pitfalls. These tips include topic-specific help as well as tips for improving exam performance.
- **Tasks to tackle.** It is important to check your understanding of the topics covered in this book on a regular basis. 'Tasks to tackle' have been set to help you do this. Once you have attempted the tasks, check your answers against those provided at the back of the book.
- **Practice makes perfect.** These exam-style questions are designed to further assess your learning and understanding. Complete these questions as you progress through each main topic area (try to do this without referring to the text answers or your own notes). Solutions are provided at the back of the book for you to check your understanding.

CD-ROM

The enclosed CD-ROM provides a selection of exam-style questions for you to tackle. These are followed by suggested answers and examiner comments. It also includes a worksheet with answers and some frequently asked questions to give you an idea of what to expect in your final exam.

The specification

The AQA AS PE course is assessed in two units. Unit 1 is entitled '**Opportunities for, and the effects of, leading a healthy and active lifestyle**'. It is assessed in a 2-hour written exam,

which counts for 60% of your AS marks. The exam paper is divided into two sections. Section A contains six structured questions, each worth 12 marks. There are two questions from each of the three specification areas of Unit 1 — Applied exercise physiology, Skill acquisition and Opportunities for participation. All questions are compulsory. Section B comprises one question applying theoretical knowledge to a practical scenario. This question is also worth 12 marks. It is set from Unit 2 theory but is assessed via the Unit 1 exam. It is important to write in continuous prose when answering this question, and to check your spelling, punctuation and grammar, as the quality of language is taken into account.

Unit 2 is called '**Analysis and evaluation of physical activity as a performer and/or in adopted roles**'. You are assessed on your ability to perform, analyse and evaluate the execution of core skills and techniques in isolation and in structured practice in two out of three roles. The three roles to select from are performer, coach and official. This unit counts for 40% of your AS mark.

As each topic area in Unit 1 is equally weighted, it is advisable to spend a similar amount of time studying each of the three theory sections. Each of these is covered in detail in this book. If you find certain topics more difficult than others, you might need to allocate a little more time to them, but try not to 'over-focus' on them. Similarly, do not concentrate on the topics that you already understand and most enjoy, as all are equally likely to be covered in the exam paper.

Unit 2 covers the theory linked to fitness and training and to the teaching and practice of skills. You will experience a lot of this theory in practical situations during lessons.

Do not be confused by the inclusion of two sections in Unit 2. All the marks for Unit 2 are awarded in Section A for your ability as a performer, official or coach/leader. Section B is the application of theoretical knowledge for effective performance. This is assessed in the last question in the Unit 1 examination, so you must revise for this.

Section A of Unit 2 involves the assessment of your ability to perform effectively in *two* of the following roles in a chosen activity from the specification:

- practical performer
- official, referee, umpire or judge
- leader or coach

You may choose to be assessed in one activity or more but the roles must be different — for example, hockey player and hockey umpire. Or you can be assessed in different activities for the two different roles — for example, as a gymnastics performer and as a rugby league referee. The assessment rubric is flexible — the essential requirement is that you undertake two *different roles*.

Role requirements are detailed in the specification. As a performer you must demonstrate the ability to perform a range of core skills and techniques, in isolation and within structured practice conditions of a non-competitive or competitive nature, according to the activity.

If you take on the role of a leader or coach, you will be assessed on your ability to analyse, modify and refine five core skills or techniques in isolation and within structured practice conditions of a non-competitive or competitive nature.

The role of official involves the assessment of your ability to officiate using fine core skills and techniques outlined in the specification, in isolation and within structured practice conditions (non-competitive and competitive).

Maximising your performance

Keeping up to date

This textbook contains topical examples but it is important to keep up to date with relevant sporting events that you can relate your studies to. For example, what is happening in the area where you live, or the school you go to, to increase participation levels among school-aged children and the local community?

This textbook gives you a sound theoretical background to build on, but reading newspapers, watching the news on television, and visiting relevant websites will keep you up to date with current policy and practice. This is particularly the case with organisations and initiatives contained in the 'Opportunities for participation' section of the specification, which is regularly reviewed with regard to mission statements and ways of achieving objectives.

In the exam

Three key elements can help you to identify the skills being tested in a particular question and to answer that question effectively:

- trigger words
- mark allocations
- knowledge of key terms

Trigger words

Some specific trigger words are used in AQA AS PE examinations. It is important that you understand the meaning of each of these words and that you answer the question appropriately.

- **Name/state/list/identify** — requires short, concise statements
- **Define/explain** — requires you to develop an answer that illustrates clearly your understanding of the topic area(s)
- **Discuss** — describe and evaluate, putting forward various opinions on a topic
- **Compare/contrast** — point out similarities and differences

If there are separate parts to a question, your answer should differentiate clearly between them. This will make your answer more examiner-friendly, which is always a good idea.

Mark allocations

Parts of questions in Section A of Unit 1 could be worth as little as 1 mark if only a short definition or explanation of a term is required — for example, **Define the term 'learning'**. Most will be worth 3–4 marks, so they do not require long, essay-style answers.

The mark allocation is indicated in brackets at the end of each part. Mark allocations are a guide to the amount of time you should spend on a question. With 120 minutes available to

score 84 marks, and no question choice to worry about, this means you have just over a minute per mark. Once you have read a question carefully and then re-read it, highlighting the key words, you should give a succinct answer that clearly attempts to answer the question set.

Section B of the Unit 1 exam is worth 12 marks. It requires you to apply knowledge of skill acquisition and fitness and training to practical scenarios. This question is awarded marks according to banded statements. Once your answer has been marked, the examiner will place it into one of the band ranges given in the mark scheme. The examiner is looking for an answer that:

- addresses all of the question
- has accessed a certain number of points from the mark scheme
- contains few errors in spelling, punctuation and grammar and uses correct technical language

It is therefore important to structure your work and to pay attention to your style of writing, as this is the one question on the Unit 1 paper where 'quality of written communication' will be assessed.

Knowledge of key terms

Build up your own glossary of terms as you progress through the topics in this textbook. This should consist of words and phrases stipulated in the Unit 1 specification. Building up your own glossary will help when you come to revise, because you will have a few pages of key terms defined clearly in ways that are meaningful to you. These will help you when you are asked to define or give the meaning of something.

Finally, don't forget to:

- **plan the length of your answers**. You will have just over a minute per mark awarded, so plan the time and amount of detail given in your answers accordingly.
- **use the trigger words and mark allocations** to identify the question demands and the degree of detail required.
- **read the question carefully**, at least twice. On the second read through, highlight key words to help you focus on the key requirements to achieve the mark allocation.
- **answer the question set**, not the one you wish was set and have revised for. Relevance is the key to success. Irrelevant answers will earn no points.
- **leave a space at the end of each question**. If you have any time left at the end of the exam, you can extend the detail of your answers without the examiner having to search for different parts of your answer.
- **avoid repetition**. Try to ensure that any points you make are sufficiently different (and relevant) to achieve marks. Students often make the number of points required by the mark allocation, thinking they will score maximum marks. This may not be the case if a point is repeated. Several alternatives are often contained within one marking point and each mark scheme point can only be awarded once.

Unit 1

Opportunities for, and the effects of, leading a healthy and active lifestyle

- Applied exercise physiology
- Skill acquisition
- Opportunities for participation

Health, exercise and fitness

What you need to know

By the end of this chapter you should be able to:
- define health and fitness and understand the relationship between them and the problems associated with their definition
- understand the effects of lifestyle choices on health and fitness
- define the health-related components of fitness — stamina, muscular endurance, strength, speed, power and flexibility
- define the skill-related components of fitness — reaction time, agility, coordination and balance

Defining fitness

Fitness is difficult to define as it means different things to different people. It can depend on individual lifestyle choices. Those who choose not to exercise regularly may think they are fit if they can run for the bus or play football in the park without getting too out of breath. On the other hand, those who have chosen an active lifestyle and exercise regularly may look at resting heart rate or heart rate recovery after exercise as an indication of fitness.

One generic definition of fitness is: **the ability to perform daily tasks without undue fatigue**. It is important to remember that these daily tasks are different for an elite performer in comparison with a non-athlete. The fitness requirements of physical activities also vary. For example, sprinting 100 m requires the body to work anaerobically with great strength, speed and power, whereas running a marathon requires good muscular and cardio-respiratory endurance.

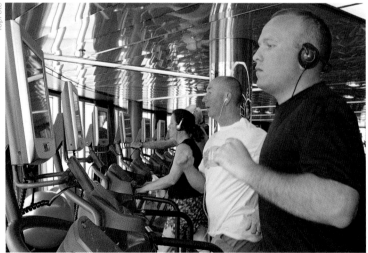

TopFoto

Many people feel the need to join a gym in order to maintain their fitness

Defining health

Physical, emotional, mental, social and spiritual well-being all influence health. There are many definitions of health. The World Health Organization defines it as: **a state of complete physical, mental and social well-being and not merely the absence of disease or infirmity.**

> ## Tasks to tackle 1.1
>
> Think of three lifestyle choices that have a negative effect on an individual's health.

This means that an elite performer who has excellent fitness may be seen as unhealthy if he/she suffers from depression. Again, lifestyle choices are important. An individual in a demanding career may have high stress levels and therefore will not be as healthy as someone in a less stressful environment.

Fitness components

Components of fitness are categorised as health-related or skill-related. The various components are shown in Figure 1.1.

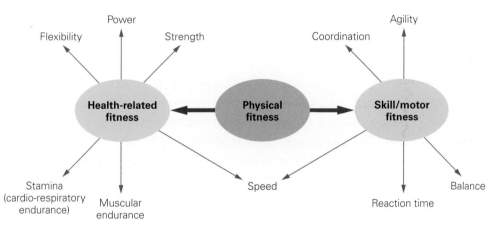

Figure 1.1 Components of fitness

Health-related components of fitness
Stamina (cardio-respiratory endurance)

Stamina is often referred to as cardio-respiratory endurance, VO_2 max or cardiovascular endurance. Whichever term is used, stamina can be defined as the ability to take in and use oxygen. This depends on three factors:

- how effectively an individual can inspire and expire
- how effective the transportation of oxygen is from the lungs to the muscles
- how well the oxygen is then used

> **Top tip**
>
> AQA classes speed as a health-related component of fitness but in some textbooks it is classed a skill/motor component of fitness.

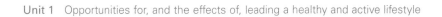

Stamina is important for participation in continuous submaximal activity, such as jogging and cycling. In team games it helps a performer to withstand fatigue.

Strength

One definition of strength is the ability to exert a force against a resistance. Different types of strength are used in sport. For example, a weightlifter needs a different type of strength to perform a maximum bench press from the strength a sprinter needs to 'explode' from the starting blocks. The three main types of strength are:

- maximum strength
- power (sometimes referred to as elastic strength)
- muscular (strength) endurance

Maximum strength is the maximum force a muscle is capable of exerting in a single voluntary contraction. It is used, for example, in weight lifting. Due to higher levels of testosterone, men have a larger muscle mass and so can exert greater maximum strength than women. Fast glycolytic fibres are important for maximum strength as they can produce more force than slow-twitch fibres.

Power (elastic strength) equates to the amount of work performed per unit of time (strength × speed). It is the ability to overcome resistance with a high speed of contraction. This can be seen in explosive events such as sprinting, throwing and hitting, where a high percentage of fast glycolytic fibres is needed for a good performance.

Muscular endurance is the ability of a muscle to perform repeated contractions and with-stand fatigue. It is important for rowers and swimmers where the same muscle action is repeated for the duration of the event. In addition, when a team game goes to extra time, the players with better muscular endurance will be in a stronger position to maintain a high level of performance. This type of strength is characterised by a high proportion of type 1 (slow oxidative) and type 2a (fast oxidative) glycolytic fibres.

Flexibility

Flexibility is the range of movement around a joint, or the resistance of a joint to movement. It is determined by the structure of the joint and the muscle elasticity. Good flexibility is important in the prevention of injury. It can also help generate faster and more forceful muscle contractions. There are two main types of flexibility:

- **Static flexibility** is the range of movement around a joint, for example around the hips when doing the splits.
- **Dynamic flexibility** is the resistance of a joint to movement, for example kicking a football without knee-joint and hip-joint resistance.

An individual's flexibility is determined by:

- the elasticity of ligaments and tendons
- the amount of stretch allowed by the surrounding muscles

- the type of joint — for example, the knee is a hinge joint allowing movement in one plane only (flexion and extension — see pp. 45–46), whereas the shoulder is a ball-and-socket joint, which allows movement in many planes (flexion, extension, abduction, adduction, rotation, horizontal adduction (flexion)/abduction (extension) and circumduction — see pp. 45–46)
- the structure of the joint — the hip and shoulder are both ball-and-socket joints but the hip joint has a deeper joint cavity and tighter ligaments to keep it more stable but less mobile than the shoulder
- the temperature of the surrounding muscle and connective tissue — warmer tissue is more flexible
- training — flexibility can decrease during periods of inactivity
- age — older people tend to be less flexible
- gender — women tend to be more flexible than men due to hormonal differences

Speed

This refers to how fast a person can move over a specified distance, or how quickly a body part can be put into motion. Speed is important in most sports: a winger in rugby needs to be a fast sprinter and a pace bowler in cricket needs to be able to move his arm quickly.

Fibre type plays a major role in terms of speed. A greater number of fast glycolytic fibres means that stimuli are received more rapidly and energy is released anaerobically, making the performer faster than someone with a greater number of slow-twitch fibres. The proportion of fast glycolytic fibres is determined genetically.

Skill-related components of fitness

Agility

Agility is the ability to move and position the body quickly and effectively while under control. The combination of speed, coordination, balance and flexibility is very important. For example, it is used in netball for catching and passing on the run, and in basketball for dribbling around opponents.

Balance

This is the ability to keep the centre of gravity over the base of support. A balance can be **static**, such as in a handstand in gymnastics, which has to be kept still, or **dynamic**, where balance is retained while in motion, for example when side-stepping in rugby to get around an opponent.

To be in a balanced position, the centre of gravity needs to be in line with the base of support. If you lower your centre of gravity, your stability increases, while if your centre of gravity starts to move near the edge of the base of support, you will start to overbalance.

Reaction time

This is the time taken from detection of a stimulus to initiation of a response, for example the time taken between the starting pistol going off and movement from the blocks, or reacting to a tennis serve.

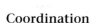

Coordination

Coordination is the ability of the motor and nervous systems to interact so that motor tasks can be performed more accurately. Examples include the hand–eye coordination required to hit a tennis ball and being able to coordinate the swing of a golf club to hit the ball correctly. Speed, precision, rhythm and fluency of execution are all important components of coordination.

Tasks to tackle 1.2

Look at the different sports performers in the table below and identify the components of fitness that are relevant to that performer. Copy the table and complete it.

	Cricketer	Gymnast	Shot-putter	Marathon runner
Stamina				
Muscular endurance				
Strength				
Speed				
Power				
Flexibility				
Reaction time				
Agility				
Coordination				
Balance				

Practice makes perfect

1 A games player needs to be agile. Identify two other components of fitness that are required by a games player and give an example of how one of these can be used in a game. *(3 marks)*

2 Define the term **power**. *(2 marks)*

3 Name two fitness components that are important for a high jumper. *(2 marks)*

4 What is meant by the terms **fitness** and **health**? *(2 marks)*

Chapter 2 *Applied exercise physiology*

Nutrition

What you need to know

By the end of this chapter you should be able to:

- identify the seven classes of food — carbohydrates, fats, proteins, vitamins, minerals, fibre and water — and highlight types of food that fall into these categories
- identify the exercise-related function of each of these types of food
- describe a balanced diet and the energy balance of food and be able to relate this to your own practical activity
- identify the difference in diet composition between endurance athletes and power athletes
- identify the percentage body fat or body composition and body mass index (BMI) as measures of nutritional suitability
- give a definition of obesity and understand the limitations in trying to define it

Nutrition and diet can contribute to a successful performance. A balanced diet is essential for optimum performance in all sporting activities. What you eat can have an effect on your health, your weight and your energy levels. Top performers place huge demands on their bodies during both training and competition. Their diet must meet their energy requirements, as well as provide nutrients for tissue growth and repair.

Nutrients

There are six groups of nutrients that should be present in any balanced diet.

Carbohydrates

There are two types of carbohydrate. Simple carbohydrates are found in fruits and are easily digested by the body. They are also present in many processed foods and anything with refined sugar added. Complex carbohydrates are found in nearly all plant-based foods, and usually take longer for the body to digest. They are most commonly found in bread, pasta, rice and vegetables.

Carbohydrate is an important energy source during activity, and it is the predominant source of energy during high-intensity exercise. Carbohydrates are stored in the muscle and liver as glycogen and transported in the form of glucose. They contain the elements carbon, hydrogen and oxygen, and store a lot of energy. It is important that carbohydrate is consumed before, during and after exercise. Carbohydrates are no longer thought of as simply fuel for

This 'food pyramid' shows the range of foods required for a healthy and balanced diet

D. Hurst/Alamy

the muscles. It is now known to be important to take into account the glycaemic index (release rate) of different carbohydrates and the consequence this has on *when* they should be consumed in relation to training.

Foods with a low glycaemic index cause a slow, sustained release of glucose to the blood, whereas as foods with a high glycaemic index cause a rapid, sharp rise in blood glucose. Suitable foods to eat 3–4 hours before exercise include beans on toast, pasta or rice with a vegetable-based sauce, breakfast cereal with milk, and crumpets with jam or honey. Suitable snacks to eat 1–2 hours before exercise include fruit smoothies, cereal bars, fruit-flavoured yoghurt and fruit. An hour before exercise, liquid consumption appears to be more important — for example, sports drinks and cordials.

Fats

Fats are the secondary energy fuel for low-intensity, aerobic work such as jogging. Fats are made from glycerol and fatty acids. Each glycerol molecule is attached to three fatty acid molecules. Glycerol and fatty acids contain the elements carbon, hydrogen and oxygen. Fats contain a lot

> **Key term**
>
> **Glycaemic index:** a ranking of carbohydrates according to their effect on blood glucose levels

of carbon. This is why they give us so much energy. Fat is an important energy fuel during low-intensity exercise but it has to be used in combination with glycogen due to its hydrophobic quality (low water solubility), which inhibits fat metabolism. Fats are stored in the muscle as triglycerides and transported as fatty acids.

Proteins

Proteins consist of chains of chemicals called amino acids. They are important for tissue growth and repair and to make enzymes, hormones and haemoglobin. Generally, proteins provide energy when glycogen and fat stores are low. However, during strenuous activity or sustained periods of exercise, proteins in the muscles may start to be broken down to provide energy.

Vitamins

Vitamins are needed for muscle and nerve functioning, tissue growth and the release of energy from foods. Over-consumption of vitamins does not have any beneficial effects as they cannot be stored in the body and excess amounts are excreted through urine.

Minerals

Minerals assist in bodily functions. For example, calcium is important for strong bones and teeth, and iron helps form haemoglobin, which is needed for the transport of oxygen and therefore to improve stamina levels. Minerals tend to be dissolved by the body as ions and are called electrolytes. These facilitate the transmission of nerve impulses and enable effective muscle contraction, both of which are important during exercise. It is important to get the right balance. Too much sodium (contained in salt) can result in high blood pressure. As with vitamins, excessive consumption is unlikely to enhance performance.

Fibre

Good sources of fibre include wholemeal bread and pasta, nuts, seeds, fruit, vegetables and pulses. Fibre is important during exercise as it can slow down the time it takes the body to break down food, which results in a slower, more sustained, release of energy.

Water

Water constitutes up to 60% of a person's body weight and is essential for good health. It carries nutrients to cells in the body and removes waste products. It also helps to control body temperature. When an athlete starts to exercise, production of water increases (water is a by-product of the aerobic system). We also lose a lot of water through sweat. The volume of water lost depends on the external temperature, the intensity and duration of the exercise and the volume of water consumed before, during and after exercise. Water is important to maintain optimal performance. Sports drinks such as Lucozade Sport and Gatorade can be used to boost glucose levels before and after competition, while water rehydrates during competition.

Dehydration is common among sports performers, especially in hot climates. Symptoms of mild dehydration are headaches and fatigue.

A balanced diet

A balanced diet should contain around 15% protein, 30% fat and 55% carbohydrate. For athletes in training, the percentage of carbohydrates should be increased. Sports nutritionists recommend:

- 10–15% proteins
- 20–25% fats
- 60–75% carbohydrates

However, endurance training makes performers such as marathon runners better at metabolising fats. This means that their fat intake needs to be increased.

The energy balance of food

When we take part in physical activity, the body needs energy. The amount of energy needed depends on the duration and type of activity. Energy is obtained from the body stores or from the food we eat. It is measured in calories; a calorie (cal) is the amount of heat energy required to raise the temperature of 1 g of water by 1°C. A kilocalorie (kcal) is the amount of heat required to raise the temperature of 1000 g of water by 1°C.

The basic energy requirement of the average person is generally given as 1.3 kcal per hour per kilogram of body weight. So someone who weighs 60 kg requires 1.3 × 24 (hours in a day) × 60 = 1872 kcal per day.

The energy requirement increases during exercise to 8.5 kcal per hour for each kilogram of body weight. So in a 1-hour training session the performer needs an extra 8.5 × 1 × 60 kg = 510 kcal.

The total energy requirement of this performer can be calculated by adding the basic energy requirement (1872 kcal) to the extra energy needed for a 1-hour training session (510 kcal): 1872 + 510 = 2382 kcal.

What should you eat before a competition?

To achieve optimal performance in sport it is essential to be well fuelled and well hydrated. The importance of a pre-competition meal should not be understated. It should be eaten 3–4 hours before competing because the food needs to be digested and absorbed in order to be useful. The meal needs to be high in carbohydrate, low in fat and moderate in fibre, to aid digestion (foods high in fat, protein and fibre tend to take longer to digest). High levels of carbohydrate will keep the blood glucose levels high throughout the competition/performance. Suggestions for pre-competition food are:

- chicken breast without skin (preferably poached)
- vegetable-based sauce
- two carbohydrate sources such as brown rice and wholemeal pasta
- unglazed vegetables
- salad, without dressing
- selection of fresh fruit (plenty of bananas)
- fresh fruit salad and yoghurt
- scrambled eggs, bacon, baked beans and fresh wholemeal toast
- porridge, Special K, muesli
- drinks: still water, orange juice, apple juice

Diet: endurance athlete versus power athlete

The body's preferred fuel for any endurance sport is muscle glycogen. If glycogen breakdown exceeds its replacement, glycogen stores become depleted. This results in fatigue and the inability to maintain the intensity of training. In order to replenish and maintain glycogen stores, an endurance athlete needs a diet rich in carbohydrates. Most research suggests that endurance athletes need to consume at least 6–10 grams of carbohydrate per kilogram of body weight per day. Water is also essential, to avoid dehydration.

Some endurance athletes manipulate their diet to maximise aerobic energy production. One method is **glycogen loading** (often called carbo-loading). Six days before an important competition the performer eats a diet high in protein and fats for 3 days and exercises at a relatively high intensity to burn off any existing glycogen stores. This is followed by 3 days of a diet high in carbohydrates and some light training. The theory is that by totally depleting glycogen stores they can then be increased by up to two times the original amount.

In general, endurance athletes require more carbohydrates than power athletes because they exercise for longer periods of time and need more energy. Proteins are very important for power athletes. Not getting enough protein leads to muscle breakdown. Proteins are necessary for tissue growth and repair.

Tasks to tackle 2.1

Copy and complete the table below with suggestions for a diet for an 18-year-old long-distance runner weighing 60 kg who trains five times a week, each session lasting 2 hours.

Energy requirements without exercise (per week)	
Energy requirements including exercise (per week)	
% carbohydrates	
% fats	
% proteins	
Suggested meals	

Body fat composition

This is the physiological make-up of an individual in terms of the distribution of lean body mass and body fat. On average, men have less body fat (15%) than women (25%).

Your percentage body fat can be estimated by the skinfold test, which measures the thickness of the skin at specific parts of the body. The total of these measurements is compared with a 'norms' table. Alternatively, the bioelectrical impedance method involves passing a small electrical current through the body to generate an estimate of body fat.

Body composition has an important role in sport. Excess body fat can lead to health problems such as cardiovascular disease, and any exercise requires more energy, since more weight has to be moved around. It is generally agreed that less body fat means a better performance. There are exceptions: some sports have specific requirements for large amounts of fat, for example the defensive linesman in American football and sumo wrestlers.

In most team games, however, excess body fat affects the performers' ability to move around the court or field and increases the onset of fatigue during the game.

Body mass index (BMI)

Body mass index or (BMI) takes into account body composition. To calculate BMI, a person's weight in kilograms is divided by his/her height (in metres) squared.

$$BMI = \frac{\text{weight (kg)}}{\text{height (m)} \times \text{height (m)}}$$

For example, for a person weighing 75 kg who is 1.80 m:

$$BMI = \frac{75}{1.80 \times 1.80} = 23.15$$

Table 2.1 Body mass index classification

BMI	Classification
<19	Underweight
19–25	Normal
26–30	Overweight
30–40	Obese
>40	Morbidly obese

BMI classifications vary but Table 2.1 is representative of most literature.

Obesity and limitations of definition

Definitions of obesity vary. In general, obesity is an excess proportion of total body fat, usually due to energy intake being greater than energy output. Obesity carries an increased risk of heart disease, hypertension, high blood cholesterol, stroke and diabetes. It increases stress on the joints and limits flexibility. There are also psychological problems associated with being obese.

An individual is considered to be obese when his/her body weight is 20% or more above normal weight, or when a male accumulates 25% and a female 35% total body fat. The body mass index can also be used as a measure of obesity. An individual is considered obese when his/her BMI is over 30.

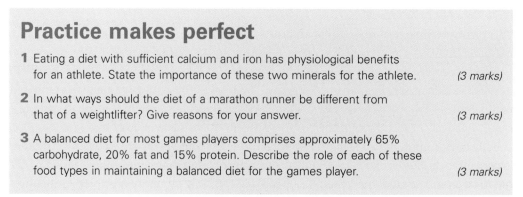

Practice makes perfect

1 Eating a diet with sufficient calcium and iron has physiological benefits for an athlete. State the importance of these two minerals for the athlete. *(3 marks)*

2 In what ways should the diet of a marathon runner be different from that of a weightlifter? Give reasons for your answer. *(3 marks)*

3 A balanced diet for most games players comprises approximately 65% carbohydrate, 20% fat and 15% protein. Describe the role of each of these food types in maintaining a balanced diet for the games player. *(3 marks)*

Chapter 3

Applied exercise physiology

Pulmonary function

What you need to know

By the end of this chapter you should be able to:

- describe the mechanics of breathing at rest and during exercise
- identify the different lung volumes and capacities and interpret them from a spirometer trace giving values at rest and during exercise
- describe the gaseous exchange process at the alveoli and muscles
- explain the principles of diffusion and the importance of partial pressures
- explain the difference in oxygen and carbon dioxide content between alveolar air and pulmonary blood
- explain how exercise can have an effect on the dissociation of oxygen from haemoglobin at the tissues (Bohr shift)
- explain how breathing is controlled (understanding the importance of carbon dioxide in this process)

The body needs a continuous supply of oxygen to produce energy. When we use oxygen to break down food to release energy, carbon dioxide is produced as a waste product and the body must remove this. Respiration, therefore, is the taking in of oxygen and the removal of carbon dioxide. It includes:

- ventilation — getting the air into and out of the lungs
- external respiration — gaseous exchange between the lungs and the blood
- transport of gases
- internal respiration — exchange of gases between the blood in the capillaries and the body cells
- cellular respiration — the metabolic reactions and processes that take place in a cell to obtain energy from fuels such as glucose (this is covered at A2)

The structure of the respiratory system

The lungs are found in the thorax. They are protected by the ribcage and separated from the abdomen by the diaphragm muscle. Each lung is surrounded by a pleura, a double membrane containing lubricating pleural fluid (see Figure 3.1). The right lung is slightly larger than the left and has three lobes; the left lung has two lobes.

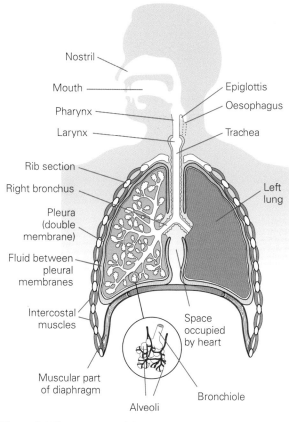

Figure 3.1 The structure of the respiratory system

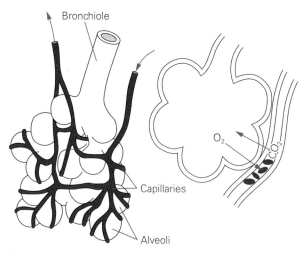

Figure 3.2 The alveoli

Air is drawn into the body through the nose, where it is warmed, humidified and filtered by a thick mucous membrane. It then passes through the pharynx and on to the larynx (voice box). The epiglottis covers the opening of the larynx to prevent food from entering the lungs. The air moves on to the trachea (windpipe). This is approximately 10 cm long and is held open by rings of cartilage. Mucus and ciliated cells line the trachea and filter the air. The trachea divides into the right and left bronchi. Air moves through the bronchi, which subdivide into secondary bronchi feeding each lobe of the lung. These get progressively thinner and branch into bronchioles, which lead into the alveolar air sacs.

The alveoli (Figure 3.2) are responsible for the exchange of gases between the lungs and the blood. Their structure is designed to help gaseous exchange. A dense capillary network supplies them with oxygen. Their walls are extremely thin (only one cell thick) and together they create a huge surface area (about the size of a tennis court in total) to allow for a greater uptake of oxygen.

The mechanics of breathing

Air moves from areas of high pressure to areas of low pressure. The greater the pressure difference, the faster air flows. This means that in order to get air into the lungs (inspiration), the pressure needs to be lower inside the lungs than in the air we are breathing. To get air out (expiration), the pressure needs to be higher in the lungs than in the air we are breathing.

Inspiration

Inspiration increases the volume of the thoracic cavity through contraction of the muscles surrounding the lungs. The diaphragm contracts and flattens while the external intercostals contract and pull the ribs up and out (Figure 3.3(a)). This reduces the pressure of air in the lungs.

Expiration

Expiration decreases the volume of the thoracic cavity. The diaphragm and external intercostals relax. This increases the pressure of air in the lungs, forcing air out (Figure 3.3(b)). At rest, expiration is a passive process.

Tasks to tackle 3.1

Rearrange the following words to show the correct order of the passage of air:

larynx → nose → trachea → pharynx → alveoli → bronchioles → bronchi

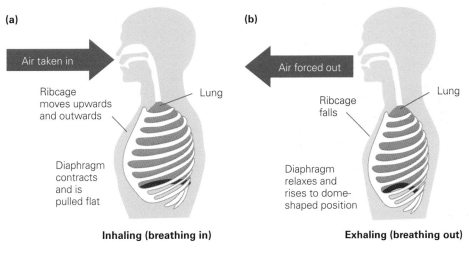

(a)

Air taken in

Ribcage moves upwards and outwards

Lung

Diaphragm contracts and is pulled flat

Inhaling (breathing in)

(b)

Air forced out

Ribcage falls

Lung

Diaphragm relaxes and rises to dome-shaped position

Exhaling (breathing out)

Figure 3.3 The mechanics of breathing

Breathing during exercise

During exercise, more muscles are involved because air needs to be forced in and out of the lungs much more quickly. The extra inspiratory muscles are the sternocleidomastoid, which lifts the sternum, and the scalenes and pectoralis minor, which help to lift the ribs. The extra expiratory muscles are the internal intercostals, which pull the ribs down and in and the abdominal muscles, which push the diaphragm up.

Lung volumes and capacities

At rest we inspire and expire approximately 0.5 litres of air per breath. The volume of air inspired or expired per breath is referred to as the tidal volume. The volume of air inspired or expired per minute is the minute ventilation and can be calculated by multiplying the number of breaths taken per minute (approximately 12) by the tidal volume:

number of breaths (per min) × tidal volume = minute ventilation

12 × 0.5 = 6 litres

At rest we still have the ability to breathe in and breathe out more air than just the tidal volume. This extra amount of air inspired is the inspiratory reserve volume (IRV); the extra amount expired is the expiratory reserve volume (ERV).

Exercise affects these lung volumes. More oxygen is required, so tidal volume needs to increase, but this reduces the ability to breathe in or out an extra amount of air, so IRV and ERV decrease (see Table 3.1).

Figure 3.4 is a spirometer trace showing an individual's lung volumes.

Top tip Look at the definition of tidal volume in Table 3.1 — *or* is a key word.

Table 3.1 Lung volumes

Lung volume or capacity	Definition	Average value at rest (litres)	Change during exercise
Tidal volume	Volume of air breathed in *or* out per breath	0.5	Increase
Inspiratory reserve volume	Volume of air that can be forcibly inspired after a normal breath	3.1	Decrease
Expiratory reserve volume	Volume of air that can be forcibly expired after a normal breath	1.2	Slight decrease
Residual volume	Volume of air that remains in the lungs after maximum expiration	1.2	No change
Vital capacity	Volume of air forcibly expired after maximum inspiration in one breath	4.8	Slight decrease
Minute ventilation	Volume of air breathed in or out per minute	6	Huge increase
Total lung capacity	Vital capacity + residual volume	6	Slight decrease

Tasks to tackle 3.2

To help you understand inspiratory reserve volume try the following:
- Take a normal breath in (tidal volume) and hold it.
- Now take another breath in until your lungs feel full. This is your inspiratory reserve volume.

To help you understand expiratory reserve volume try the following:
- Breathe out normally (tidal volume) and hold it.
- Now breathe out further as much as you can. This is your expiratory reserve volume.

Work out what happens to these volumes during exercise. This time the initial breath in and out needs to be much deeper as breathing is both quicker and deeper during exercise.

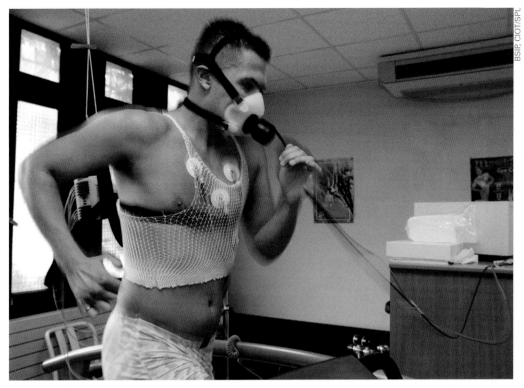

BSIP, CIOT/SPL

Lung volumes and levels of gases can be measured at different levels of activity, using specialist apparatus

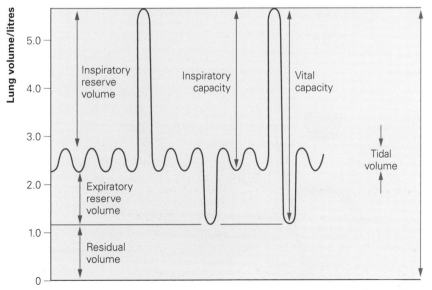

Figure 3.4 Spirometer trace of respiratory air

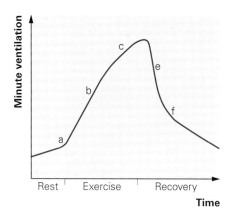

Figure 3.5 Minute ventilation response to maximal exercise

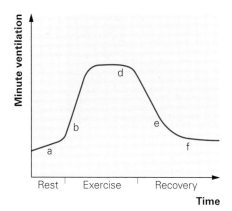
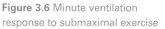

Figure 3.6 Minute ventilation response to submaximal exercise

Changes in pulmonary ventilation occur during different types of exercise. As you would expect, the more demanding the physical activity, the more breathing increases to meet the extra oxygen demand. This is illustrated in Figures 3.5 and 3.6.

a = anticipatory rise

b = sharp rise in minute ventilation

c = slower increase

d = steady state

e = rapid decline in minute ventilation

f = slower recovery as body systems return to resting levels

Gaseous exchange at the lungs

Gaseous exchange at the lungs (external respiration) is concerned with the replenishment of oxygen in the blood and the removal of carbon dioxide. Partial pressure is often used when describing the gaseous exchange process. All gases exert a pressure. Oxygen makes up a part of air (approximately 21%), so it exerts a partial pressure. Since gases flow from areas of high pressure to areas of low pressure, it is important that, as oxygen moves from the alveoli to the blood and then to the muscle, the partial pressure of oxygen of each is successively lower.

The partial pressure of oxygen in the alveoli (105 mmHg) is higher than the partial pressure of oxygen in the capillary blood vessels (40 mmHg). This is because the working muscles remove oxygen, so its concentration in the blood is lower and therefore so is its partial pressure. The difference between any two pressures is referred to as the diffusion (concentration) gradient and the steeper this gradient, the faster the diffusion. Oxygen diffuses from the alveoli into the blood until the pressure is equal in both.

The movement of carbon dioxide occurs in the same way but in the reverse order, from the muscle to the blood to the

Key term

Partial pressure: the pressure exerted by an individual gas when it exists within a mixture of gases.

Table 3.2 Percentages of gases and water content in inspired and expired air

	Inspired air (%)	Expired air at rest (%)	Expired air during exercise (%)
Oxygen	21	16.4	15
Carbon dioxide	0.03	4.0	6
Nitrogen	79	79.6	79
Water vapour	Varies	Saturated	Saturated

alveoli. The partial pressure of carbon dioxide in the blood entering the alveolar capillaries is higher (45 mmHg) than that in the alveoli (40 mmHg), so carbon dioxide diffuses from the blood into the alveoli until the pressure is equal in both.

> **Top tip**
> Remember that the diffusion of gases at the alveoli is helped by the alveolar structure. Alveoli are only one cell thick, so there is a short diffusion pathway; they have a vast surface area, which facilitates diffusion; and they are surrounded by a vast network of capillaries.

Gaseous exchange at the tissues (internal respiration)

For diffusion to occur, the partial pressure of oxygen must be lower in the tissues than in the blood. The partial pressure of oxygen in the capillary membranes surrounding the muscle is 40 mmHg and in the blood it is 105 mmHg. This allows oxygen to diffuse from the blood into the muscle until equilibrium is reached.

Conversely, the partial pressure of carbon dioxide is lower in the blood (40 mmHg) than in the tissues (45 mmHg), so again diffusion occurs and carbon dioxide moves into the blood to be transported to the lungs.

> **Key terms**
> **A-VO$_2$ diff:** the difference between the oxygen content of arterial blood and that of venous blood.
> **Diffusion gradient (concentration gradient):** explains how gases flow from areas of high concentration to areas of low concentration. The steeper the gradient (i.e. the greater the difference between concentration levels), the faster diffusion occurs.

Arterio-venous oxygen difference

The arterio-venous difference (A-VO$_2$ diff) is the difference in the oxygen content of the arterial blood arriving at the muscles and the venous blood leaving the muscles. At rest, the arterio-venous difference is low because the muscles do not require much oxygen. During exercise, however, the muscles need more oxygen from the blood, so the arterio-venous difference is high. This increase in A-VO$_2$ diff affects gaseous exchange at the alveoli, due to the high concentration of carbon dioxide and lower concentration of oxygen returning to the heart in the venous blood. This increases the diffusion gradient for both gases. Training also increases the arterio-venous difference because trained performers can extract more oxygen from the blood.

Figure 3.7 highlights the differences in the partial pressure of oxygen and carbon dioxide in the alveoli, in the blood and in muscle cells.

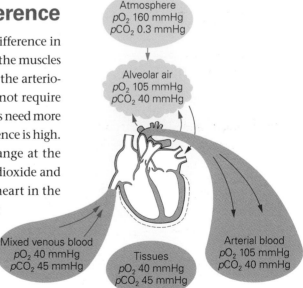

Figure 3.7 Partial pressures of oxygen and carbon dioxide in the respiratory system

Transportation of oxygen

During exercise, oxygen diffuses into the capillaries supplying the skeletal muscles. Three percent dissolves in plasma and 97% combines with haemoglobin to form oxyhaemoglobin. Fully saturated haemoglobin carries four oxygen molecules. Haemoglobin is fully saturated when the partial pressure of oxygen in the blood is high, for example in the alveolar capillaries of the lungs. At the tissues, oxygen dissociates from haemoglobin because of the lower partial pressure of oxygen that exists there.

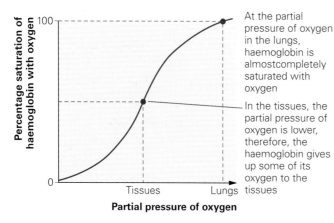

At the partial pressure of oxygen in the lungs, haemoglobin is almostcompletely saturated with oxygen

In the tissues, the partial pressure of oxygen is lower, therefore, the haemoglobin gives up some of its oxygen to the tissues

Figure 3.8 The oxyhaemoglobin dissociation curve

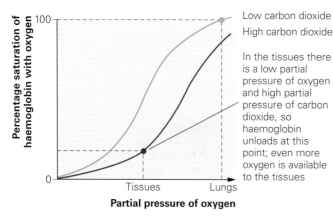

Low carbon dioxide

High carbon dioxide

In the tissues there is a low partial pressure of oxygen and high partial pressure of carbon dioxide, so haemoglobin unloads at this point; even more oxygen is available to the tissues

Figure 3.9 The Bohr shift

Bohr effect: the reduction in the affinity of haemoglobin for oxygen owing to an increase in blood carbon dioxide and a decrease in pH.

Key term

The relationship of oxygen and haemoglobin is often represented by the oxyhaemoglobin dissociation curve (Figure 3.8).

At the partial pressure of oxygen in the lungs, haemoglobin is almost completely saturated with oxygen. In the tissues, the partial pressure of oxygen is lower and therefore the haemoglobin gives up some of its oxygen to the tissues.

Under certain conditions, haemoglobin gives up some of its oxygen more readily and the S-shaped curve shifts to the right (Figure 3.9). This is important during exercise when there is a greater demand for oxygen. These conditions are:

- an increase in temperature of the blood and muscle
- a decrease in the partial pressure of oxygen in the muscle during exercise, increasing the oxygen diffusion gradient
- an increase in partial pressure of carbon dioxide during exercise, increasing the carbon dioxide diffusion gradient
- an increase in acidity during exercise. This is caused by the increase in carbon dioxide in the blood, which results in an increase in the concentration of hydrogen ions in the blood ($CO_2 + H_2O \rightleftharpoons H^+ + HCO_3^-$), lowering the pH (the Bohr effect).

Control of ventilation

The nervous system can increase or decrease the rate, depth and rhythm of breathing. The respiratory centre located in the medulla oblongata of the brain controls breathing. An increased concentration of carbon dioxide in the blood stimulates the respiratory centre to increase respiratory rate.

Top tip

A question on control of ventilation may refer to how an increase in carbon dioxide can affect breathing.

The respiratory centre has two main areas. The inspiratory centre is responsible for inspiration and expiration. The expiratory centre stimulates the expiratory muscles during exercise, when stretch receptors detect changes in the rate and depth of breathing.

The inspiratory centre sends out impulses via the phrenic nerve to the inspiratory muscles. When the stimulus stops, expiration occurs.

During exercise, conditions in the body change. These changes are detected by:
- chemoreceptors, which detect changes in pH — blood acidity increases as a result of an increase in the plasma concentration of carbon dioxide and lactic acid production
- baroreceptors, which detect an increase in blood pressure
- proprioceptors, which detect movement

An impulse is sent to the respiratory centre and then down the phrenic nerve to the inspiratory muscles. As a result the rate, depth and rhythm of breathing increase.

During exercise, the lungs are stretched more. Stretch receptors prevent over-inflation of the lungs by sending impulses to the expiratory centre and then down the intercostal nerve to the expiratory muscles so that expiration occurs.

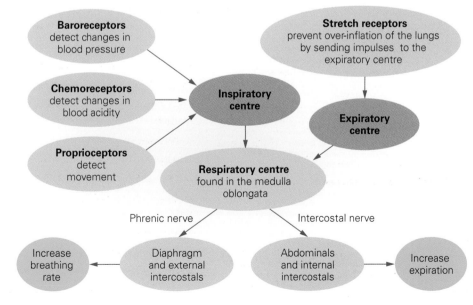

Figure 3.10 Control of ventilation

Practice makes perfect

1 During exercise the demand for oxygen by the muscles increases.
How is breathing rate controlled to meet these demands?   *(4 marks)*

2 What does the term arterio-venous difference (A-VO$_2$ diff) mean?
Why does it increase during exercise?   *(2 marks)*

3 During exercise, the oxyhaemoglobin curve shifts to the right. Explain the
causes of this shift and identify the effect that this has on oxygen delivery
to the muscles.   *(4 marks)*

4 Define tidal volume. Identify what happens to tidal volume during exercise.   *(2 marks)*

5 Performance in sporting activities is influenced by gas exchange and
oxygen delivery. Explain how oxygen diffuses from the lungs into the blood
and how it is transported to the tissues.   *(4 marks)*

6 Describe the mechanisms of breathing at rest.   *(3 marks)*

Transport of blood gases: the vascular system

What you need to know

By the end of this chapter you should be able to:
- explain pulmonary and systemic circulation related to the various blood vessels (arteries, arterioles, capillaries, venules and veins)
- describe the venous return mechanism
- understand how blood is redistributed during exercise (vascular shunt)
- describe how oxygen and carbon dioxide are transported in the blood, and understand the roles of haemoglobin and myoglobin
- explain what is meant by blood pressure and velocity and relate these terms to specific blood vessels

Transportation of blood around the body

The vascular system is made up of blood vessels that carry blood through the body. These blood vessels deliver oxygen and nutrients to the body tissues and take away waste products such as carbon dioxide. Together with the heart and lungs, the blood vessels ensure that the muscles have an adequate supply of oxygen during exercise in order to cope with the increased demand for energy.

There are two types of circulation (Figure 4.1):
- the **pulmonary** circulation takes deoxygenated blood from the heart to the lungs and oxygenated blood back to the heart
- the **systemic** circulation carries oxygenated blood to the body from the heart and returns deoxygenated blood from the body to the heart

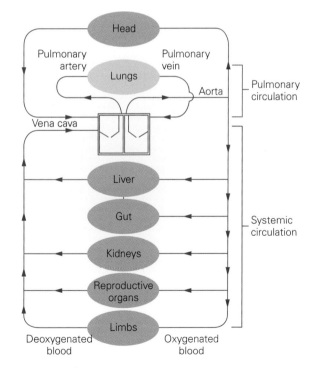

Figure 4.1 Circulation of blood

Blood vessels

The vascular system consists of five different types of blood vessel that carry the blood from the heart, distribute it around the body and then return it to the heart. Arteries carry blood away from the heart. The heart beat pushes blood through the arteries by surges of pressure and the elastic arterial walls expand with each surge, which can be felt as a pulse in the arteries near the surface of the skin. The arteries then branch off and divide into smaller vessels called arterioles, which in turn divide into microscopic vessels called capillaries. These have a single cell layer of endothelium cells and are only wide enough to allow one red blood cell to pass through at a given time. This slows the blood flow, which allows time for the exchange of substances with the tissues to take place by diffusion. There is a dense capillary network surrounding the tissues and this creates a large surface area for diffusion to take place. Blood then flows from the capillaries to the venules, which increase in size and eventually form veins, which return the blood under low pressure to the heart.

To summarise, the order in which the blood flows through the vascular system is:

heart → arteries → arterioles → capillaries → venules → veins → heart

Structure of the blood vessels

Arteries, arteriole, venules and veins all have a similar structure (Figure 4.2). Their walls consist of three layers:

- The **tunica externa** (adventitia) is the outer layer, which contains collagen fibres. This wall needs to be elastic in order to stretch and withstand large fluctuations in blood volume.
- The **tunica media** is the middle layer, which is made up of elastic fibres and smooth muscle. The elastic fibres stretch when blood is forced into the arteries during ventricular systole. When they recoil they smooth out the flow of blood and push it along the arteries. The smooth muscle can contract in the walls of the smaller arteries and arterioles, which ensures that the amount of blood flowing to different organs varies according to demand.
- The **tunica interna** is made up of thin epithelial cells that are smooth and reduce friction between the blood and the vessel walls.

All blood vessels have features that adapt them to their particular functions. These are summarised in Table 4.1.

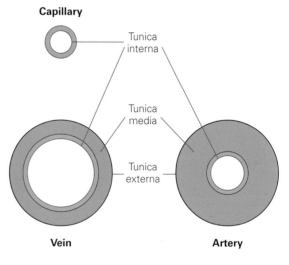

Figure 4.2 Structure of blood vessels

Table 4.1 Blood vessel adaptations

Feature	Artery	Capillary	Vein
Tunica externa (outer layer)	Present	Absent	Present
Tunica media (middle layer)	Thick with many elastic fibres	Absent	Thinner and less elastic than an artery
Tunica interna (inner layer)	Present	Present	Present
Size of lumen	Small	Microscopic	Large
Valves	Absent	Absent	Present

The venous return mechanism

Venous return is the transport of blood to the right side of the heart via the veins. Up to 70% of the total blood volume is contained in the veins at rest. This provides a large reservoir of blood, which is returned rapidly to the heart when needed.

The heart can only pump out as much blood as it receives, so cardiac output is dependent on venous return. A rapid increase in venous return enables a significant increase in stroke volume and therefore cardiac output. Veins have a large lumen and offer little resistance to blood flow. Blood pressure is low by the time blood enters the veins. This means that active mechanisms are needed to help venous return. These include:

- the **skeletal muscle pump** (Figure 4.3). When muscles contract and relax, they change shape. This change in shape means that the muscles press on nearby veins, causing a pumping effect and squeezing blood towards the heart.
- the **respiratory pump**. When muscles contract and relax during the inspiration and expiration process, pressure changes occur in the thoracic and abdominal cavities. These pressure changes compress the nearby veins and assist the flow of blood back to the heart.
- **valves**. It is important that blood in the veins only flows in one direction. The valves ensure that this happens. Once the blood has passed through the valves, they close to prevent the blood flowing back.
- **smooth muscle**. There is a thin layer of smooth muscle in the walls of the veins. This helps to squeeze blood back towards the heart.

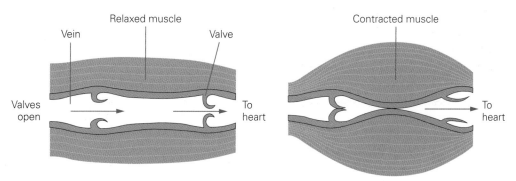

Figure 4.3 The skeletal muscle pump

Venous return must be maintained during exercise to ensure that the skeletal muscles receive enough oxygen to meet the demands of the activity. At rest, the valves and the smooth muscle in veins are sufficient to maintain venous return. During exercise, the demand for oxygen is greater and the heart beats faster, so the vascular system has to help out too. The skeletal muscle pump and the respiratory pump ensure venous return is maintained. This is possible during exercise because the skeletal muscles are constantly contracting and the breathing rate is elevated. These mechanisms need to be maintained immediately after exercise. Performing an active cool-down keeps the skeletal muscle pump and respiratory pump working, and thus prevents the blood from pooling.

The vascular shunt

During exercise, blood flow to the skeletal muscles increases to meet the increase in oxygen demand. This redirection of blood flow to the areas where it is most needed is known as shunting, or the **vascular shunt** mechanism (Figure 4.4).

> **Key term**
>
> **Vascular shunt mechanism:** the redistribution of cardiac output (blood flow).

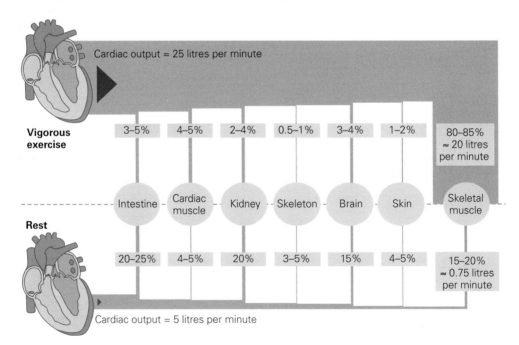

Figure 4.4 The vascular shunt

Sports performers should not eat within an hour of competition. Eating results in blood being redirected to the stomach to aid digestion. This would affect performance because less oxygen would be available for the muscles. Blood flow to the brain remains constant to ensure that brain function is maintained.

The control of blood flow

The **vasomotor centre** is located in the medulla oblongata of the brain. It controls both blood pressure and blood flow. During exercise, chemical changes such as increases in carbon dioxide and lactic acid are detected by chemoreceptors. Higher blood pressure is detected by baroreceptors. These receptors stimulate the vasomotor centre, which redistributes blood flow through vasodilation and vasoconstriction.

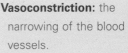

Vasoconstriction: the narrowing of the blood vessels.
Vasodilation: the widening of the blood vessels.

Vasodilation increases blood flow; **vasoconstriction** decreases blood flow. During exercise, the working muscles require more oxygen, so vasodilation occurs in the arterioles supplying the skeletal muscles, increasing blood flow and bringing in the much-needed oxygen. At the same time, vasoconstriction occurs in the arterioles supplying non-essential organs, such as the intestines and the liver.

Redirection of blood flow also occurs through stimulation of the sympathetic nerves located in the tunica media of the blood vessel. When stimulation by the sympathetic nerves decreases, vasodilation occurs and when sympathetic stimulation increases, vasoconstriction occurs.

Precapillary sphincters also aid blood redistribution. These are tiny rings of muscle located at the opening of capillaries. When they contract, blood flow is restricted through the capillary and when they relax, blood flow is increased. During exercise, the precapillary sphincters of the capillary networks supplying skeletal muscle relax. This increases blood flow, which in turn helps to saturate the tissues with oxygen.

Redistribution of blood is important to:
- increase the supply of oxygen to the working muscles
- remove waste products such as carbon dioxide and lactic acid from the muscles
- ensure more blood goes to the skin during exercise to regulate body temperature and get rid of heat through radiation, evaporation and sweating
- direct more blood to the heart, since it is a muscle that requires extra oxygen during exercise

Oxygen and carbon dioxide in the vascular system

Oxygen plays a major role in energy production. A reduction in the amount of oxygen in the body has a detrimental impact on performance. During exercise, when oxygen diffuses into the capillaries supplying the skeletal muscles, 3% dissolves in plasma and 97% combines with haemoglobin to form oxyhaemoglobin. At the tissues, oxygen dissociates from haemoglobin because of the lower pressure of oxygen that exists there. In the muscle, oxygen is stored by **myoglobin**. This has a high affinity for oxygen and stores the oxygen until it can be transported from the capillaries to the mitochondria. The mitochondria are the sites in the muscle where aerobic respiration takes place.

Myoglobin: a protein that stores oxygen in the muscle.

Carbon dioxide is transported around the body in the following ways:

- 70% is transported in the blood as hydrogen carbonate (bicarbonate) ions. The carbon dioxide produced by the muscles as a waste product diffuses into the bloodstream where it combines with water to form carbonic acid. Carbonic acid is a weak acid that dissociates into hydrogen carbonate ions.
- 23% combines with haemoglobin to form carbaminohaemoglobin.
- 7% dissolves in plasma.

An increase in the level of carbon dioxide results in an increase in blood and tissue acidity. This is detected by chemoreceptors, which send impulses to the medulla. Heart rate, breathing rate and transport increase so that more carbon dioxide is exhaled and the arterial blood levels of both oxygen and carbon dioxide are maintained.

Blood pressure and blood flow

Blood pressure is the force exerted by the blood against the blood vessel wall and is often referred to as:

blood flow × resistance

Ejection of the blood by the ventricles contracting creates a high-pressure pulse of blood, which is known as systolic pressure. The lower pressure as the ventricles relax is the diastolic pressure.

Blood pressure is measured at the brachial artery (in the upper arm) using a sphygmomanometer. A typical reading at rest is 120/80 mm Hg (millimetres of mercury). The first figure (120) is the systolic pressure; the lower figure (in this case 80) is the diastolic pressure.

Blood pressure varies in the different blood vessels and depends largely on the distance of the blood vessel from the heart (Figure 4.5):

- artery — high and in pulses
- arteriole — not quite as high

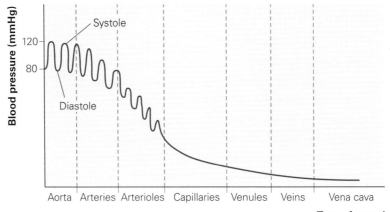

Figure 4.5 Blood pressure as a function of vessel type

- capillary — pressure drops throughout the capillary network
- vein — low

Blood velocity

The velocity of blood flow changes as the blood passes from one type of blood vessel to another. The velocity depends on the total cross-sectional area of the vessel. The smaller the cross-sectional area, the faster the blood flows.

Although the capillaries are the smallest of the blood vessels, the fact that there are so many of them means that their total cross-sectional area is much greater than that of the aorta. This

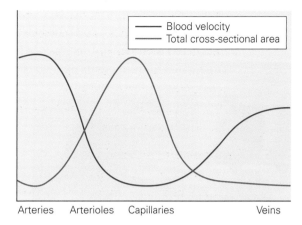

Figure 4.6 Relationship between blood velocity and vessel cross-sectional area

means that the flow of blood is slower in the capillaries and this allows time for efficient exchange of substances with the tissues. This relationship between blood velocity and cross-sectional area of the different blood vessels is shown in Figure 4.6.

Exercise and its effects on blood pressure

Changes in blood pressure occur during exercise and these depend on the type and intensity of the exercise. During aerobic exercise, systolic pressure increases due to an increase in stroke volume and cardiac output. Vasodilation can cause a reduction in blood pressure because of the decrease in resistance to blood flow that occurs. However, the significant increases in stroke volume and cardiac output outweigh this. Diastolic pressure remains constant during aerobic exercise.

During isometric work, diastolic pressure increases due to increased resistance in the blood vessels. This is because during isometric work the muscle remains contracted, causing constant compression on the blood vessels, which results in an additional resistance to blood flow in the muscles and therefore an increase in pressure.

Tasks to tackle 4.1

Copy and complete the table below to show what happens to the systolic pressure of an 18-year-old PE student on a 40-minute training run.

Blood pressure changes	Before exercise	During exercise	Recovery

Control of blood pressure

The vasomotor centre controls blood pressure. Baroreceptors located in the aortic and carotid arteries detect increases and decreases in blood pressure and send an impulse to the vasomotor centre located in the medulla oblongata (Figure 4.7).

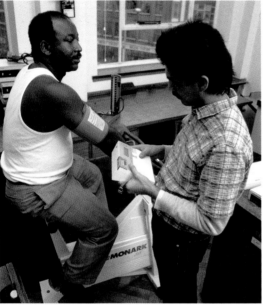

Blood pressure is measured using a sphygmomanometer

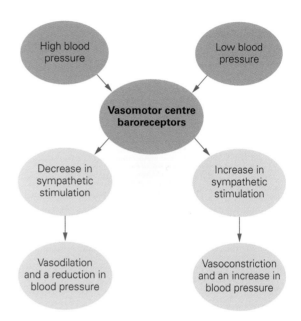

Figure 4.7 Control of blood pressure

Practice makes perfect

1 Describe the mechanisms that are used to return blood to the heart. *(3 marks)*

2 Why does blood flow to the brain remain the same at rest and during exercise? *(2 marks)*

3 Why should an athlete not eat within 1 hour before competition? *(3 marks)*

4 How is carbon dioxide transported in the blood? *(2 marks)*

5 Explain how blood is redistributed to the working muscles. *(3 marks)*

6 Give an average blood pressure reading and identify what happens to blood pressure during exercise. *(2 marks)*

Chapter 5 *Applied exercise physiology*

Cardiac function

What you need to know

By the end of this chapter you should be able to:

- describe the stages of the cardiac cycle and understand how it is linked to the conduction system
- give definitions of cardiac output, stroke volume and heart rate, and explain the relationship between them
- understand Starling's law of the heart
- explain heart rate range in response to exercise and describe the hormonal and nervous effects on heart rate
- explain the role of blood carbon dioxide in changing heart rate
- explain cardiovascular drift
- describe the concept of cardiac hypertrophy and how it leads to bradycardia/athlete's heart

Structure of the heart

The heart is a muscular, cone-shaped organ and is approximately the size of a clenched fist. It is located in the chest between the lungs and is protected by the rib cage. The main purpose of the heart is to pump blood around the body.

Chambers of the heart

The heart is divided into two parts by a muscular wall called the septum (Figure 5.1). Each part contains an atrium and a ventricle. The atria are smaller than the ventricles because all they do is push blood into the ventricles. This does not require much force so they have thinner muscular walls. The ventricles have much thicker muscular walls as they need to contract with greater force in order to push blood

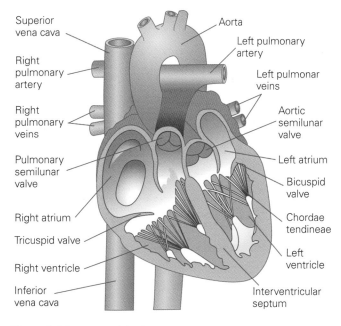

Figure 5.1 Structure of the heart

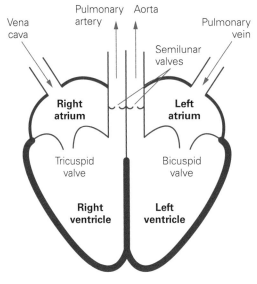

Figure 5.2 The blood vessels of the heart

out of the heart. The left side of the heart has the thickest walls as it needs to pump blood all around the body, whereas the right side pumps deoxygenated blood to the lungs, which are in close proximity to the heart.

Blood vessels of the heart

The **vena cava** carries deoxygenated blood from the body to the right atrium. The **pulmonary artery** carries deoxygenated blood from the right ventricle to the lungs. The **pulmonary vein** delivers oxygenated blood from the lungs to the left atrium. The **aorta** carries oxygenated blood from the left ventricle to the body (Figure 5.2).

For the heart to work effectively, it requires a good blood supply. This is provided by the coronary artery, which carries oxygenated blood. Deoxygenated blood is removed by the veins of the heart into the right atrium through the coronary sinus.

Tasks to tackle 5.1

Describe the journey taken by a red blood cell from the gastrocnemius in the calf where it is carrying deoxygenated blood until it leaves the aorta transporting oxygenated blood.

Valves of the heart

There are four main valves in the heart that regulate blood flow by ensuring it moves in only one direction. They open to allow blood to pass through and then close to prevent backflow. The tricuspid valve is located between the right atrium and the right ventricle. The bicuspid valve lies between the left atrium and the left ventricle. The semilunar valves are located between the right ventricle and the pulmonary artery and between the left ventricle and the aorta respectively.

The conduction system

Blood needs to flow through the heart in a controlled manner, in through the atria and out through the ventricles. Contraction of heart muscle is described as being **myogenic** (it creates its own impulse). An electrical impulse originates in the sinoatrial node (pacemaker) of the heart (Figure 5.3). This electrical signal then spreads through the heart in what is often described as a wave of excitation (similar to a Mexican wave).

From the sinoatrial node, the electrical signal spreads through the walls of the atria, causing them to contract and forcing blood into the ventricles. The signal then passes through the atrioventricular node, found in the atrioventricular septum. The atrioventricular node delays the transmission of the cardiac impulse for approximately 0.1 seconds to enable the atria to contract fully before ventricular contraction begins. The electrical signal then passes down through some specialised fibres, which form the bundle of His. This is located in the septum separating the two ventricles. The bundle of His branches out into two bundle branches and then into smaller bundles called Purkyne fibres, which spread throughout the ventricles, causing them to contract.

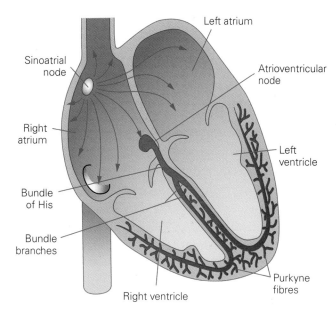

Figure 5.3 The conduction system of the heart

The cardiac cycle

Diastole: the relaxation phase of the heart.
Systole: the contraction phase of the heart.

The cardiac cycle describes the emptying and filling of the heart. It involves a number of stages. The diastole phase is when the chambers are relaxing and filling with blood. The systole phase is when the heart contracts and forces blood either around the heart or out of the heart to the lungs and the body. Each complete cardiac cycle takes approximately 0.8 seconds. The diastole phase lasts 0.5 seconds and the systole phase lasts for 0.3 seconds. The cardiac cycle is summarised in Table 5.1.

Table 5.1 The cardiac cycle

Stage	Action	Result
Atrial systole	Atrial walls contract	Blood is forced through the bicuspid and tricuspid valves into the ventricles.
Atrial diastole	Atrial walls relax	Blood enters the right atrium via the vena cava and the left atrium via the pulmonary vein but cannot pass into the ventricles as the tricuspid and bicuspid valves are closed.
Ventricular systole	Ventricular walls contract	Pressure of blood opens the semilunar valves and blood is ejected into the pulmonary artery to the lungs and into the aorta to the body. The tricuspid and bicuspid valves close.
Ventricular diastole	Ventricular walls relax	Blood enters from the atria (passive ventricular filling, not due to atrial contraction). The semilunar valves are closed.

Link between the cardiac cycle and the conduction system

The cardiac cycle describes the flow of blood through the heart during one heartbeat. Since the heart generates its own electrical impulses, this flow of blood is controlled via the conduction system.

Cardiac dynamics

Stroke volume

Stroke volume is the amount of blood pumped out by the left ventricle in each contraction. The average resting stroke volume is approximately 70 ml.

Stroke volume is determined by:

- venous return — the volume of blood returning to the heart via the veins. If venous return increases, stroke volume will also increase (i.e. if more blood enters the heart then more blood is pumped out).
- the elasticity of the cardiac fibres — this is concerned with the degree of stretch of cardiac tissue during the diastole phase of the cardiac cycle. The more the cardiac fibres stretch, the greater the force of contraction. A greater force of contraction can increase stroke volume. This is called **Starling's law.**
- the contractility of the cardiac tissue (myocardium) — the greater the contractility of the cardiac tissue, the greater the force of contraction. This results in an increase in stroke volume. Stroke volume is also affected by an increase in the ejection fraction (the percentage of blood pumped out of the left ventricle per beat). An average value is 60% but it can increase by up to 85% following a period of training.

$$\text{ejection fraction} = \frac{\text{stroke volume}}{\text{end diastolic volume}} \times 100$$

Key terms

Cardiac output: the amount of blood pumped out of the left ventricle per minute.

Ejection fraction: the percentage of blood pumped out of the left ventricle per beat.

Starling's law: when stroke volume increases in response to an increase in the volume of blood filling the left ventricle

(end diastolic volume). The increased volume of blood stretches the ventricular wall, causing cardiac muscle to contract more forcefully.

Stroke volume: the amount of blood pumped out by the left ventricle per beat.

Venous return: blood returning to the heart via the veins.

Heart rate

Heart rate is the number of times the heart beats per minute. The average resting heart rate is approximately 72 beats per minute. The fitter an individual, the lower the heart rate. For example, Miguel Indurain, an elite cyclist, had a resting heart rate of only 28 beats per minute.

Cardiac output

Cardiac output is the amount of blood pumped out by the left ventricle per minute. It is equal to stroke volume multiplied by heart rate.

$$\text{cardiac output } (Q) = \text{stroke volume} \times \text{heart rate}$$
$$Q = 70 \times 72$$
$$Q = 5040 \text{ ml (5.04 litres)}$$

If heart rate or stroke volume increases, then cardiac output will also increase.

Heart rate range in response to exercise

Heart rate increases with exercise but how much it increases depends on the intensity of the exercise. Heart rate increases in direct proportion to exercise intensity until it reaches a maximum. Maximum heart rate can be approximated by subtracting the performer's age from 220. For example, a 17-year-old will have a maximum heart rate of around 203 beats per minute.

Figures 5.4 and 5.5 illustrate the changes in heart rate during maximal exercise such as sprinting and submaximal exercise such as jogging.

In Figures 5.4 and 5.5:

a = the **anticipatory rise** due to the hormonal action of adrenaline, which stimulates the sinoatrial node to make the heart beat faster and stronger

b = a sharp rise in heart rate at the beginning of exercise due mainly to anaerobic work

c = the heart rate continuing to rise due to maximal workloads stressing the anaerobic system

d = a steady state as the athlete is able to meet the oxygen demand required for the activity (reaching a plateau)

e = a rapid decline in heart rate as soon as the exercise stops, because there is a decrease in the demand for oxygen by the working muscles

f = a slow recovery as the body systems return to resting levels (but the heart rate remains elevated to rid the body of waste products such as lactic acid).

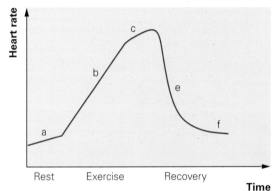

Figure 5.4 Heart rate response to maximal exercise

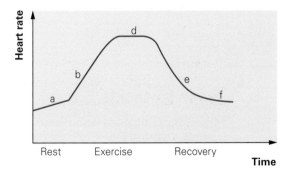

Figure 5.5 Heart rate response to submaximal exercise

Always label your graphs clearly.

Top tip

Cardiac output in response to exercise

Regular aerobic training results in hypertrophy of the cardiac muscle — the heart muscle gets physically bigger and stronger. This has an important effect on stroke volume and heart rate, and therefore on cardiac output. A bigger heart means that more blood can be pumped out of the left ventricle per beat (i.e. stroke volume increases). In more complex language, the end diastolic volume of the ventricle increases. If the ventricle can contract with more force and thus push out more blood, the resting heart rate will decrease. This is known as bradycardia.

This increase in stroke volume and decrease in resting heart rate means that cardiac output at rest remains unchanged. However, this is not the case during exercise. An increase in heart rate coupled with an increase in stroke volume results in an increase in maximum cardiac output. Cardiac output increases as the intensity of exercise increases until maximum exercise capacity is achieved and a plateau is reached (Figure 5.6).

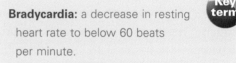

Bradycardia: a decrease in resting heart rate to below 60 beats per minute.

Table 5.2 shows the differences in cardiac output (to the nearest litre) in a trained and untrained individual both at rest and during exercise. The individual in this example is aged 18 so the maximum heart rate is 202 beats per minute.

Table 5.2 Effect of training on cardiac output

	Stroke volume/ml	Heart rate/ beats per min	Q/litres
Untrained, at rest	70	72	5
Untrained, during exercise	120	202	24
Trained, at rest	85	60	5
Trained, during exercise	170	202	34

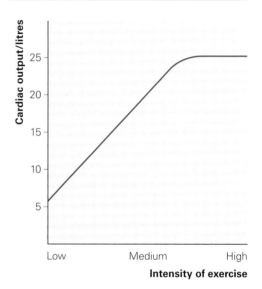

Figure 5.6 Cardiac output versus exercise intensity

Tasks to tackle 5.2

Measuring heart rate response to varying intensities of workload

1 Work in pairs and get the passive partner to take and record heart rate values.

2 Note your heart rate while you are resting for a 10-second count.

3 Record your heart rate immediately before the exercise commences for a 10-second count.

4 Commence your choice of submaximal exercise for a period of 3 minutes.

5 Take heart rate values for a 10-second pulse count:
- at the end of the 3 minutes of exercise
- every minute during the recovery phase until your heart rate has returned to its resting value prior to exercise

6 Once your heart rate has returned to its resting value, repeat the investigation but increase the workload to medium intensity.

7 Repeat the investigation at high intensity.

8 Collate your results in a table similar to the one below.

Intensity of workload	Resting heart rate	Heart rate prior to exercise	Heart rate at end of exercise	Heart rate during recovery					
				1	2	3	4	5	6
Low									
Medium									
High									

9 Represent your results graphically.

This increase in cardiac output has huge benefits for the trained individual as he/she can transport more blood and therefore more oxygen to the working muscles. In addition, when the body starts to exercise, the distribution of blood flow changes. This means that a much higher proportion of blood passes to the working muscles and less passes to non-essential organs such as the intestine. The amount of blood passing to the kidneys and the brain remains unaltered.

Stroke volume in response to exercise

Stroke volume increases as exercise intensity increases but only up to 40–60% of maximum effort. Once a performer reaches this point, stroke volume levels out (Figure 5.7). One explanation is that the increased heart rate near maximum effort results in a shorter diastolic phase. The ventricles have less time to fill up with blood, so they cannot pump as much out.

Control of heart rate

Heart rate increases during exercise to ensure that the working muscles receive more oxygen. The heart generates its own impulses from the sinoatrial node but the rate at which these cardiac impulses are fired is controlled by two main mechanisms:
- neural
- hormonal

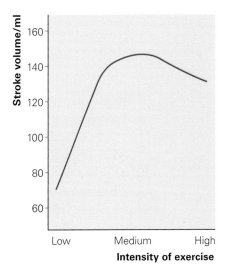

Figure 5.7 Stroke volume as a function of exercise intensity

Neural control mechanism

The autonomic nervous system comprises the sympathetic system and the parasympathetic system. The sympathetic system stimulates the heart to beat faster; the parasympathetic system returns the heart to its resting level. The cardiac control centre located in the medulla oblongata of the brain coordinates these two systems. The cardiac control centre is stimulated by chemoreceptors, baroreceptors and proprioceptors.

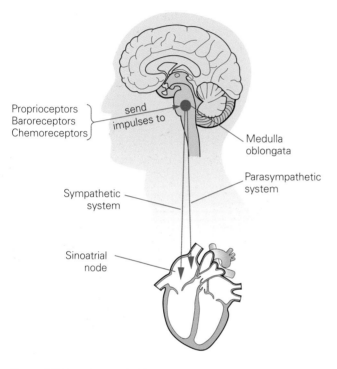

Proprioceptors
Baroreceptors
Chemoreceptors

send impulses to

Medulla oblongata

Parasympathetic system

Sympathetic system

Sinoatrial node

Figure 5.8 Neural control of heart rate

During exercise, chemoreceptors detect increases in carbon dioxide and lactic acid and decreases in oxygen. The role of blood carbon dioxide is important in controlling heart rate. Baroreceptors detect increases in blood pressure; proprioceptors detect increases in muscle movement. These receptors send impulses to the cardiac control centre, which then sends an impulse through the sympathetic nervous system or cardiac accelerator nerve to the sinoatrial node to increase heart rate.

When exercise stops, carbon dioxide levels, blood pressure and muscle movement all decrease. This is detected by the receptors, which send impulses to the cardiac control centre. An impulse is then sent through the parasympathetic system or paravagus nerve, which stimulates the sinoatrial node and heart rate decreases. This process is summarised in Figure 5.8.

Top tip

Don't be vague. Tell the examiner what the receptors detect — for example, chemoreceptors detect increases in carbon dioxide.

Hormonal control mechanism

Adrenaline and noradrenaline are stress hormones that are released by the adrenal glands. Exercise causes a stress-induced adrenaline response. This results in:

- stimulation of the sinoatrial node, which results in an increase in both the speed and force of contraction
- an increase in blood pressure due to the constriction of blood vessels
- an increase in blood glucose levels — glucose is used by the muscles for energy

Cardiovascular drift

It used to be thought that exercising at a steady level led to the body reaching a steady state, with heart rate remaining constant. However, new research has shown that heart rate does not remain the same but instead increases slowly. This is called **cardiovascular drift**. It is characterised by a progressive decrease in stroke volume and arterial blood pressure, together with a progressive rise in heart rate. It occurs during prolonged exercise in a warm environment despite the intensity of the exercise remaining the same. It is suggested that cardiovascular drift occurs because when we sweat a portion of the lost fluid volume comes from the plasma volume. The decrease in plasma volume reduces venous return and stroke volume. Heart rate increases to compensate and maintain constant cardiac output. To minimise cardiovascular drift, it is important to maintain high fluid consumption before and during prolonged exercise.

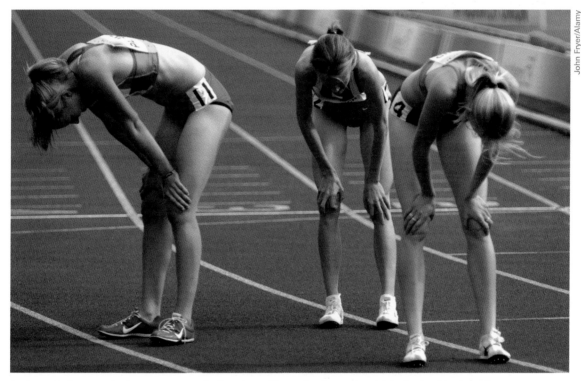

John Fryer/Alamy

At the end of a race, the heart rate soon declines but will remain elevated to rid the body of lactic acid

Effects of training on the heart

If you perform continuous, fartlek or aerobic interval training over a period of time, physiological adaptations take place that make the initial training sessions appear very easy.

Key term

VO$_2$ max: the maximum amount of oxygen that can be taken in and used by the body in 1 minute.

This is because VO_2 max improves due to changes made by the body. Some of these changes affect the heart, which becomes much more efficient:

- **Athlete's heart** is a common term for an enlarged heart caused by repeated strenuous exercise. Due to the demands of exercise, the chambers of the heart enlarge, which allows them to fill with more blood during the diastolic phase of the cardiac cycle. This results in an increase in the volume of blood that can be pumped out per beat, so the heart has to contract less frequently.
- **Hypertrophy** of the myocardium means that the heart gets bigger and stronger. This results in bradycardia (a decrease in resting heart rate) and an increase in stroke volume.
- Maximum cardiac output increases but cardiac output at rest and during submaximal exercise remains the same.
- Increased capillarisation of the heart muscle increases the efficiency of oxygen diffusion into the myocardium.
- Increased contractility — resistance or strength training causes an increase in the force of heart contractions due to a thickening of the ventricular myocardium. This increases stroke volume and ejection fraction, as a higher percentage of blood is pumped.

Practice makes perfect

1 During exercise, heart rate increases to meet the extra oxygen demand required by the muscles. Explain how the increasing level of carbon dioxide in the blood raises heart rate. *(3 marks)*

2 What effect would a 6-month period of aerobic training have on the heart of a soccer player? *(3 marks)*

3 Just before the start of an 800 m race, an athlete will experience a change in heart rate. What change occurs in the athlete's heart rate and why does this happen? *(2 marks)*

4 Explain the terms **bradycardia** and **athlete's heart**. *(2 marks)*

5 Define the terms **cardiac output** and **stroke volume** and explain the relationship between them. *(3 marks)*

6 What are the effects of a period of training on *resting* stroke volume and cardiac output? *(2 marks)*

Chapter 6 Applied exercise physiology

Analysis of movement

What you need to know

By the end of this chapter you should be able to:
- analyse shoulder and elbow actions in push-ups, overarm throwing and forehand racket strokes
- analyse hip, knee and ankle actions in running, kicking, jumping and squats

Analysing these sporting actions requires knowledge of:
- the type of joint, articulating bones and joint actions
- the main agonists and antagonists
- types of muscle contraction — concentric, eccentric, isometric

You need to be able to:
- relate the movements occurring at joints to planes and axes
- identify the three classes of lever and give examples of their use in the body in relation to the specified sporting actions
- explain the relationship of levers to effective performance, with reference to mechanical advantages and disadvantages and range and speed of movement

The skeleton

The skeleton (Figure 6.1, p. 42) is made up of 206 bones. It comprises the axial skeleton, which is made up of the skull, the vertebral column, the sternum and the ribs, and the appendicular skeleton, which comprises the shoulder girdle, the hip girdle, and the bones of the arms, hands, legs and feet.

The skeleton has a number of functions:
- Support — the skeleton provides a rigid framework to the body.
- Levers — the bones act as a lever system, allowing movement.
- Attachment — the skeleton provides suitable sites for the attachment of muscles.
- Protection — the skeleton protects the internal organs. For example, the cranium protects the brain and the ribcage protects the heart and lungs.
- Blood cell production — both red and white blood cells are produced within the bone marrow. Red blood cells are produced at the ends of long bones, such as the femur in the leg and the humerus in the arm.
- Shape — the skeleton gives the body shape.

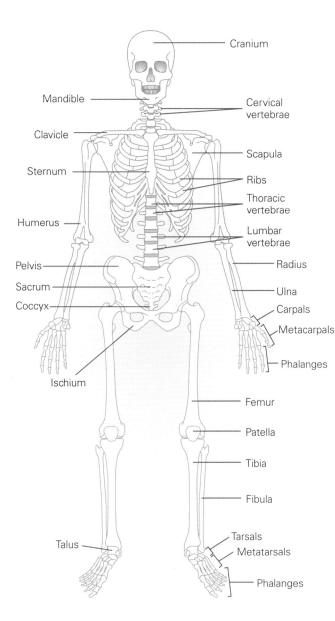

Cranium

Mandible

Cervical vertebrae

Clavicle

Sternum

Scapula

Ribs

Thoracic vertebrae

Humerus

Lumbar vertebrae

Pelvis

Radius

Sacrum

Ulna

Coccyx

Carpals

Metacarpals

Phalanges

Ischium

Femur

Patella

Tibia

Fibula

Tarsals

Talus

Metatarsals

Phalanges

Figure 6.1 The human skeleton

You will not be asked to label a skeleton in the exam but you do need to know the names of the bones that articulate at the ankle, knee, hip, shoulder and elbow.

Top tip

Joints

The skeleton is a framework connected by joints. Joints are necessary for muscles to lever bones, thus creating movement. A joint is formed where two or more bones meet. Joints are classified by how much movement they allow. There are three types of joint:

- fibrous
- cartilaginous
- synovial

Fibrous joints allow no movement at all — they are completely fixed. There is no joint cavity and the bones are held together by fibrous, connective tissue. Examples of this type of joint can be found in the cranium, the facial bones and the pelvic girdle.

Cartilaginous joints occur where the bones are separated by cartilage. They allow only a slight amount of movement. Examples of this type of joint are the ribs joining the sternum and the vertebrae joining to form the spine.

Synovial joints allow movement in one or more directions and are the most common of the three joints. These joints have a fluid-filled cavity surrounded by an articular capsule. Hyaline or articular cartilage is found at the ends of the bones where they come into contact with each other. This prevents friction between the articulating bones. There are six types of synovial joint:

- ball-and-socket
- hinge
- pivot
- condyloid
- gliding
- saddle

Ball-and-socket joints allow the most movement. They are formed by the round head of one bone fitting into the cup-shaped capsule of the connecting bone. The hip (Figure 6.2) and the shoulder (Figure 6.3) are ball-and-socket joints.

Hinge joints usually allow movement in one plane only, owing to the shape of the bones that make up the joint. Examples of this type of joint are the ankle, the knee and the elbow (Figures 6.4–6.6).

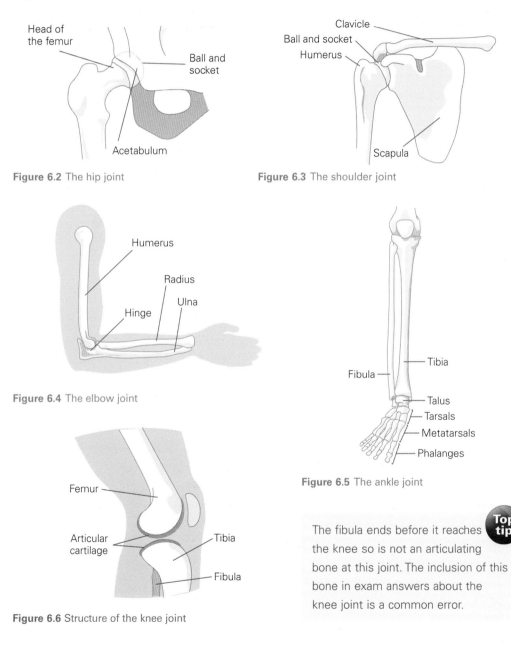

Figure 6.2 The hip joint

Figure 6.3 The shoulder joint

Figure 6.4 The elbow joint

Figure 6.5 The ankle joint

Figure 6.6 Structure of the knee joint

Top tip

The fibula ends before it reaches the knee so is not an articulating bone at this joint. The inclusion of this bone in exam answers about the knee joint is a common error.

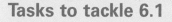

Tasks to tackle 6.1

The specification requires knowledge of the hip, shoulder, elbow, knee and ankle joints only. Use the labelled skeleton on p. 42 to work out the articulating bones for these joints, and complete a table similar to the one below.

Joint	Joint type	Articulating bones
Ankle	Hinge	
Knee	Hinge	
Hip	Ball and socket	
Shoulder	Ball and socket	
Elbow	Hinge	

Pivot joints allow rotational movement only, where the head of one bone fits into a notch on another. The atlas and axis vertebrae in the neck (cervical 1 and 2) and the joint between the radius and the ulna are pivot joints.

Condyloid joints are similar to hinge joints but instead of allowing movement in just one plane they allows sideways motion too. The dome-shaped surface of one bone fits into the hollow-shaped depression of the other. Examples of this type of joint are found in the wrist.

Gliding joints allow slight movement in all directions between two flat surfaces. Examples are found between the small bones of the wrist (metacarpals) and feet (metatarsals) as well as the articular processes of the vertebrae.

The bones that make up a saddle joint have a concave and a convex surface, which are placed together. The thumb joint is an example.

Planes and axes

To help explain movement, the body can be viewed as having a series of imaginary slices running through it. These are referred to as planes of movement (Figure 6.7).

- The sagittal (median) plane is a vertical plane that divides the body into right and left sides.

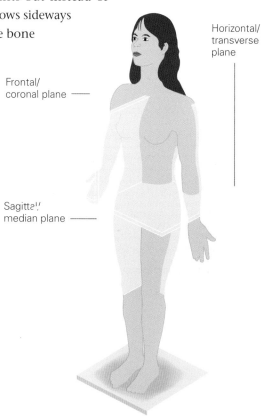

Frontal/coronal plane

Horizontal/transverse plane

Sagittal/median plane

Figure 6.7 Planes of movement

- The frontal (coronal) plane is also a vertical plane but this divides the body into front and back.
- The transverse plane is a horizontal plane that divides the body into upper and lower halves.

A body, or body part, will move in one or more of these planes, depending on the action being performed. In a full twisting somersault, for example, the gymnast will move in all three planes.

There are three axes of movement (imaginary lines through the body) about which rotation occurs:

- The transverse axis runs from side to side through the body.
- The sagittal axis runs from front to back.
- The vertical axis runs from top to bottom.

Most movements occurring at joints are related to both axes and planes. For example, flexion and extension occur in a sagittal plane about a transverse axis, rotation occurs in a transverse plane about a vertical axis and abduction and adduction occur in a frontal plane about a sagittal axis.

Types of movement

Movement in a sagittal plane

Flexion involves a *decrease* in the angle that occurs around a joint. For example, bending the arm at the elbow causes the angle between the radius and the humerus to decrease (Figure 6.8).

Extension involves an *increase* in the angle that occurs around a joint. For example, straightening the knee causes an increase in the angle between the femur and the tibia (Figure 6.9).

Plantarflexion is a term used solely for the ankle joint. It involves bending the foot downwards, away from the tibia (standing on your tiptoes).

Dorsiflexion is bending the foot upwards towards the tibia, or bending the hand backwards (Figure 6.10).

Movement in a frontal plane

Abduction is movement away from the midline of the body — for example, raising the arms out to the side, away from the body.

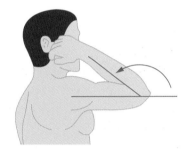

Figure 6.8 Elbow flexion

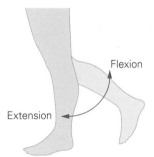

Figure 6.9 Extension and flexion of the knee

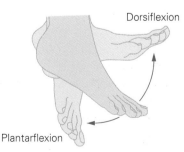

Figure 6.10 Plantarflexion and dorsiflexion

Adduction is movement towards the midline of the body — for example, lowering the arms back to the sides of the body (Figure 6.11).

Remember adduction and abduction as follows. If something is *abducted*, it is taken away. Look at the word *add*uction — think of adding the arm or leg back to the body.

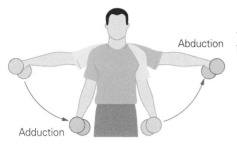

Figure 6.11 Adduction and abduction

Movement in a transverse plane

Horizontal adduction (also called horizontal flexion) is movement of the arm forward across the body at 90° to shoulder abduction. For example, raise your arm out to the side until it is parallel to the floor (abduction of the shoulder) and then move it back across the body, keeping it parallel to the floor (Figure 6.12).

Horizontal abduction (also called horizontal extension) is movement of the arm backwards across the body to shoulder abduction. For example, raise your arm forward and hold it at 90° (flexion of the shoulder), then move it away from the body, keeping it parallel to the floor (Figure 6.13).

Rotation is movement of a bone about its axis. This can be inward (medial) or outward (lateral) — see Figure 6.14.

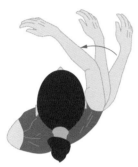

Figure 6.12 Horizontal adduction

Movement in two planes

Circumduction involves movement in the sagittal and the transverse planes, when the lower end of the bone moves around in a circle. It is a combination of flexion, extension, abduction and adduction. Circumduction occurs at the shoulder and hip joints (Figure 6.15).

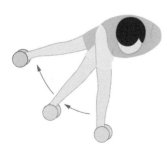

Figure 6.13 Horizontal abduction

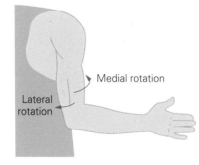

Figure 6.14 Lateral and medial rotation

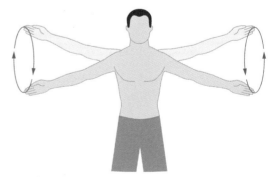

Figure 6.15 Circumduction at the shoulders

Tasks to tackle 6.2

Work out the types of movement that can take place at each joint and tick the relevant boxes to complete the table.

	Elbow	Shoulder	Hip	Knee	Ankle
Flexion					
Extension					
Abduction					
Adduction					
Rotation					
Horizontal abduction					
Horizontal adduction					
Plantarflexion					
Circumduction					
Dorsiflexion					

Muscles

There are over 600 muscles in the human body, comprising approximately 45% of the total body weight. There are three main types of muscle tissue:

- skeletal
- cardiac
- smooth

Skeletal muscle is often referred to as voluntary, striped or striated muscle (Figure 6.16). It is attached to bone and produces movement. Skeletal muscle can occur in layers, where 'deep' muscles lie below 'superficial' muscles (Figure 6.17, p. 48).

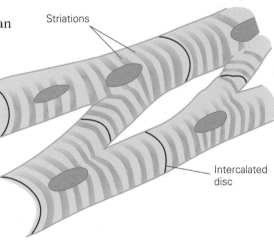

Figure 6.16 Structure of skeletal muscle

Cardiac muscle is found in the heart. It forces blood into the circulatory blood vessels, such as the aorta and the pulmonary artery. Cardiac muscle cells can only respire aerobically and therefore have the highest concentration of mitochondria. Cardiac muscle has a long rest

Table 6.1 Comparison of skeletal and cardiac muscle

Skeletal	Cardiac
Voluntary	Involuntary
Brain sends an impulse for it to contract	Myogenic – creates its own impulse
Parallel fibres	Intercalating fibres
Fewer, smaller mitochondria	More, larger mitochondria

Top tip

In terms of PE, skeletal muscle is the most important type and the one that is examined in detail.

period so that no summation occurs between contractions. This allows the heart to beat in a rhythmic manner with a rest period between contractions. This rest period prevents fatigue in the cardiac muscle.

Smooth muscle lies internally and has several functions, the main ones being to force food through the digestive system and to squeeze blood through the circulatory system via the artery and arteriole networks.

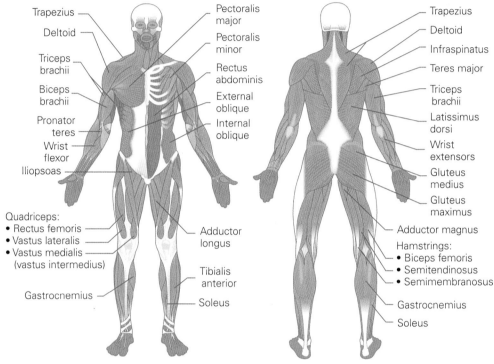

Figure 6.17 Human skeletal muscles

Actions of muscles

A joint cannot move by itself — it needs muscles to move the bones into position.

Muscles are attached to bones by tendons. The attachment of the muscle on a bone nearest the midline of the body (proximal end) is referred to as the origin. This is normally a stable, flat bone. The attachment on a bone further away from the midline of the body (distal end) is the insertion; this is the bone that the muscle moves.

When a muscle contracts, it shortens and bulges and the insertion moves closer to the origin. For example, the origin of the biceps brachii is on the scapula and the insertion is on the radius. The biceps is responsible for flexion of the elbow. When the biceps contracts, the radius moves upwards towards the shoulder, thus moving the insertion closer to the origin.

Movement at a joint usually involves several muscles. Each muscle plays a particular role so that movement can take place in an effective and controlled manner. When the muscle contracts, it is responsible for the movement that occurs and is said to be acting as an **agonist** or **prime mover**. There may be more than one agonist acting at a joint, although this depends on the type of movement that is being performed. An **antagonist** muscle is one that works in opposition to the agonist, so when the biceps brachii (the agonist) is contracting, the triceps brachii is lengthening and acting as the antagonist.

When one muscle is acting as an agonist and another is acting as the antagonist, the muscles are said to be working together as an antagonistic pair. In a flexion of the knee movement, the hamstrings are the agonist and the quadriceps are the antagonist.

As well as antagonistic muscle pairs, other muscles contract to make the joint movement stable. These are **fixator** muscles. Fixators are muscles that stabilise the origin so that the agonist can work more efficiently. For example, in the upward phase of an arm curl, the biceps brachii is the agonist, the triceps brachii is the antagonist and the deltoid is the fixator. You can feel tension in the deltoid as it helps to stabilise the shoulder joint.

> **Key terms**
>
> **Agonist:** the muscle responsible for the movement.
>
> **Antagonist:** the muscle that works in opposition to the agonist, helping to produce a coordinated movement.

> **Top tip**
>
> **Be careful.** The agonist does not automatically become the antagonist when the movement changes, for example from flexion to extension. In the downward phase of the biceps curl, most students think that the biceps is the antagonist, but it is still the agonist. It is now lengthening as it contracts in order to control the lowering of the forearm while it supports the weight.

Joints for the exam

For the AS examination, you need to know about movements of the elbow, shoulder, hip, knee and ankle joints.

The elbow joint

The elbow is a hinge joint, with the distal (far) end of the humerus articulating with the proximal (near) end of the radius and ulna (Figure 6.18). Movement can take place in one plane only, allowing only flexion and extension (Table 6.2).

Table 6.2 Movement in the elbow joint

Movement	Agonist	Plane
Flexion	Biceps brachii	Sagittal
Extension	Triceps brachii	Sagittal

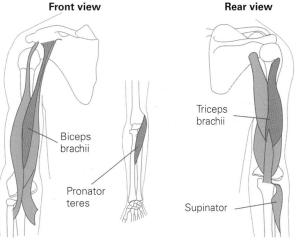

Figure 6.18 Muscles of the elbow joint

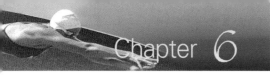

The shoulder joint

The shoulder is a ball-and-socket joint where the head of the humerus fits into a cavity on the scapula called the glenoid fossa. This type of joint allows the most movement, because of the shallowness of the joint cavity. However, its structure also makes it one of the least stable joints, so it is heavily reliant on ligaments and muscles to increase its stability (Figure 6.19 and Table 6.3).

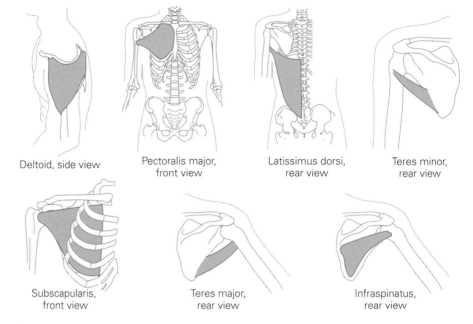

Deltoid, side view   Pectoralis major, front view   Latissimus dorsi, rear view   Teres minor, rear view

Subscapularis, front view   Teres major, rear view   Infraspinatus, rear view

Figure 6.19 Muscles of the shoulder joint

Table 6.3 Movement at the shoulder joint

Movement	Agonist	Plane
Flexion	Anterior deltoid	Sagittal
Extension	Posterior deltoid	Sagittal
Abduction	Middle deltoid	Frontal
Adduction	Latissimus dorsi	Frontal
Lateral rotation	Teres minor	Transverse
Medial rotation	Subscapularis	Transverse
Horizontal abduction	Latissimus dorsi	Transverse
Horizontal adduction	Pectoralis major	Transverse

Top tip

You need to know one muscle for each of the movements, so make it easy for yourself and learn each of the different sections of the deltoid, which covers three movements.

The hip joint

The hip is a ball-and-socket joint where the head of the femur fits into the acetabulum of the pelvis. The joint cavity for the hip is much deeper than that for the shoulder, thus making the hip more stable but less mobile. The addition of strong muscles and ligaments surrounding the hip joint decreases its mobility even more, but at the same time this makes dislocation very difficult (Figure 6.20 and Table 6.4).

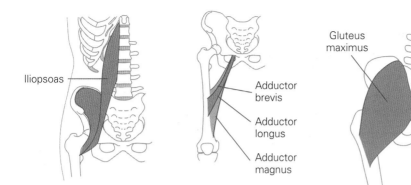

Figure 6.20 Muscles of the hip joint

The knee joint

The knee is classed as a hinge joint and so should only be able to flex and extend (Table 6.5). However, this is not strictly true as some rotation is allowed to facilitate full extension and locking of the knee. The femur articulates with the tibia (not the fibula). Strong ligaments are present in order to prevent any sideways movement. Muscles controlling the knee are shown in Figure 6.21.

Table 6.4 Movement at the hip

Movement	Agonist	Plane
Flexion	Iliopsoas	Sagittal
Extension	Gluteus maximus	Sagittal
Abduction	Gluteus medius	Frontal
Adduction	Adductors	Frontal
Lateral rotation	Gluteus maximus	Transverse
Medial rotation	Gluteus medius	Transverse

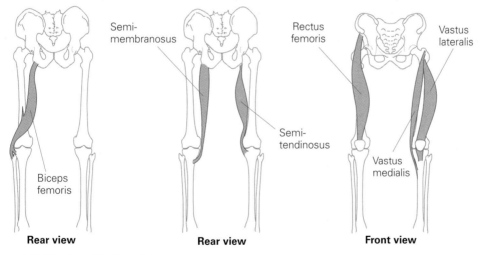

Figure 6.21 Muscles of the knee joint

Table 6.5 Movement at the knee joint

Movement	Agonist	Plane
Flexion	Hamstrings: biceps femoris, semitendinosus, semimembranosus	Sagittal
Extension	Quadriceps: rectus femoris, vastus lateralis, vastus medialis, vastus intermedius	Sagittal

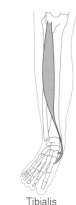

Gastrocnemius
(double-headed calf muscle)

Tibialis
anterior

Figure 6.22 Muscles of the ankle joint

The ankle joint

The ankle is a hinge joint where the articulating bones are the tibia, fibula and talus. The two main muscles that control movement in this joint are the gastrocnemius and the tibialis anterior (Figure 6.22), allowing plantarflexion and dorsiflexion respectively (Table 6.6).

Table 6.6 Movement at the ankle joint

Movement	Agonist	Plane
Plantarflexion	Gastrocnemius	Sagittal
Dorsiflexion	Tibialis anterior	Sagittal

Types of muscular contraction

A muscle can contract in three different ways, depending on the muscle action that is required:

- concentric contraction
- eccentric contraction
- isometric contraction

Concentric contraction is when the muscle shortens under tension. For example, during the upward phase of an arm curl, the biceps brachii performs a concentric contraction as it shortens to produce flexion of the elbow.

Eccentric contraction is when the muscle lengthens under tension (and does not relax). When a muscle contracts eccentrically, it acts as a brake to help control the movement of the body part during negative work. For example, when landing from a standing jump, the quadriceps muscles are performing negative work as they are supporting the weight of the body during landing. The knee joint is in the flexed position but the quadriceps muscles are unable to relax as the weight of the body ensures that they lengthen under tension.

Isometric contraction is when the muscle contracts without lengthening or shortening. The result is that no movement occurs. An isometric contraction occurs when a muscle acts as a fixator or against a resistance.

Using the biceps curl as an example (Figure 6.23):

- During the upward phase, the biceps brachii contracts to produce flexion of the elbow joint. In this situation it is performing a concentric contraction.

Concentric contraction: when a muscle shortens under tension.
Eccentric contraction: when a muscle lengthens under tension.
Isometric contraction: when a muscle is under tension but there is no visible movement.

- During the downward phase, if you put your hand on the biceps brachii you will still feel tension. This means that the muscle is not relaxing but is performing an eccentric contraction, where it lengthens under tension.
- If the weight is held still at a 90° angle, the biceps brachii is under tension although there is no movement. This is an isometric contraction.

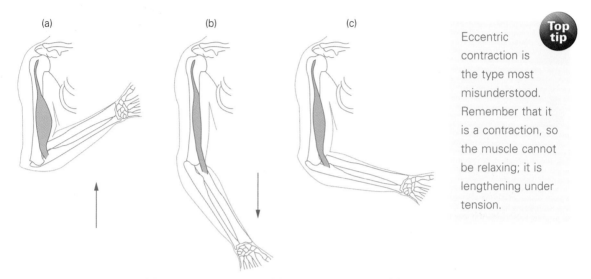

(a) (b) (c)

Top tip

Eccentric contraction is the type most misunderstood. Remember that it is a contraction, so the muscle cannot be relaxing; it is lengthening under tension.

Figure 6.23 The biceps curl: (a) concentric contraction, (b) eccentric contraction, (c) isometric contraction

Levers

A lever consists of three main components, namely a pivot (fulcrum), the weight to be moved (resistance) and a source of energy (effort or force). The skeleton forms a system of levers that allows us to move. The bones act as the levers — the joints are the fulcrums and the effort is provided by the muscles.

The main functions of a lever are:
- to increase the speed at which the body can move
- to increase the resistance that a given effort can move

Levers can be classified as:
- first-order
- second order
- third order

First-order levers are where the fulcrum is between the effort and the resistance (Figure 6.24, p. 54). First-order

Tasks to tackle 6.3

Answer the following questions for the movements involved in a press-up.

1 During the downward phase:
- What type of movement happens at the elbow joint?
- Which muscle contracts?
- What type of contraction occurs?

2 During the upward phase:
- What type of movement happens at the elbow joint?
- Which muscle contracts?
- What type of contraction occurs?

3 If the press-up is held in the downward phase:
- Which muscle feels as if it contracts?
- What type of contraction occurs?

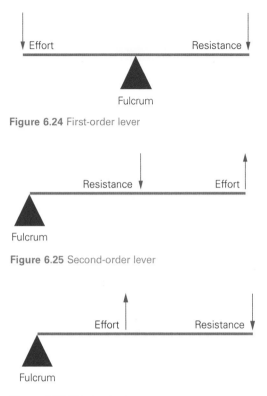

Figure 6.24 First-order lever

Figure 6.25 Second-order lever

Figure 6.26 Third-order lever

levers can increase both the effects of the effort and the speed of the body. Examples of this type can be seen in the movement of the head and neck during flexion and extension and in the action of extending the limbs.

Second-order levers are where the resistance lies between the fulcrum and the effort (Figure 6.25). This type of lever generally increases only the effect of the effort, that is, it can be used to overcome heavy loads. Plantarflexion of the ankle involves the use of a second-order lever.

Third-order levers are responsible for the majority of movements in the human body. They can increase the body's ability to move quickly, but in terms of applying force they are very inefficient. The effort lies between the fulcrum and the resistance (Figure 6.26) and can be seen in the forearm during flexion of the elbow.

Tasks to tackle 6.4

Label the fulcrum, effort and resistance in Figure 6.27.

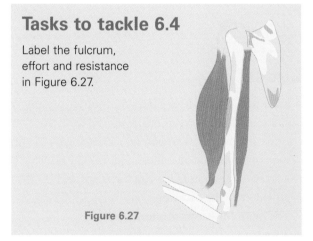

Figure 6.27

The **effort arm** or **force arm** is the shortest perpendicular distance between the fulcrum and the application of the effort (force). The **resistance arm** is the shortest perpendicular distance between the fulcrum and the resistance. The force arm and the resistance arm are shown in the third-order lever in Figure 6.28.

When the resistance arm is longer than the effort arm, the lever system is at a **mechanical disadvantage**. This means that it cannot move as heavy a load but it can move the load faster. When the effort arm is longer than the resistance arm, the lever system is at a **mechanical advantage**. This means that it can move a large load over a short distance and requires little effort.

Length of lever

Most levers in the body are third-order levers where the resistance arm is always greater than the effort arm (mechanical disadvantage). The longer the resistance arm of the lever, the greater the speed at the end of it. This means that if the arm is fully extended when bowling or passing, for example, the ball will travel with most force and at the greatest speed. The use of a cricket bat, tennis racket or golf club effectively extends the arm and allows more force to be exerted.

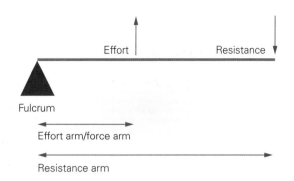

Figure 6.28 The effort arm and the resistance arm

Joint movement analysis

For the AQA specification you have to be able to perform a movement analysis of the following skills:

- shoulder and elbow action in the forehand racket stroke
- shoulder and elbow action in a throw
- elbow action in a press-up
- hip, knee and ankle action in a kick
- hip, knee and ankle action in a jump
- knee and ankle action in a squat
- hip, knee and ankle action in running

Key terms

Mechanical advantage: when the effort arm is longer than the resistance arm.

Mechanical disadvantage: when the resistance arm is longer than the effort arm.

Shoulder and elbow action in the forehand racket stroke

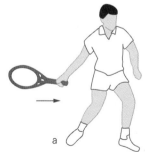
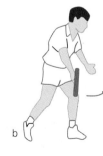
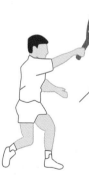
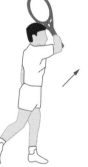

Movement	Agonist	Antagonist	Plane	Axis	Type of contraction	Lever system
a–d Shoulder action: horizontal adduction (horizontal flexion)	Pectoralis major	Latissimus dorsi	Transverse	Longitudinal	Concentric	Third order
c–d Elbow action, flexion	Biceps brachii	Triceps brachii	Sagittal	Transverse	Concentric	Third order

Shoulder and elbow action in an overarm throw

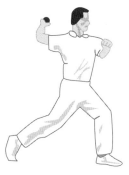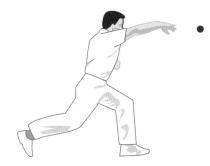

Movement	Agonist	Antagonist	Plane	Axis	Type of contraction	Lever system
Shoulder action: horizontal adduction (horizontal flexion)	Pectoralis major	Latissimus dorsi	Transverse	Longitudinal	Concentric	Third order
Elbow action: extension	Triceps brachii	Biceps brachii	Sagittal	Transverse	Concentric	First order

Elbow action in a press-up

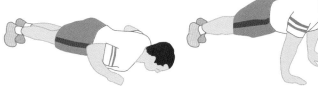

Movement	Agonist	Antagonist	Plane	Axis	Type of contraction	Lever system
Upward phase/extension	Triceps brachii	Biceps brachii	Sagittal	Transverse	Concentric	First order
Downward phase/flexion	Triceps brachii	Biceps brachii	Sagittal	Transverse	Eccentric	

Hip, knee and ankle action in a kick

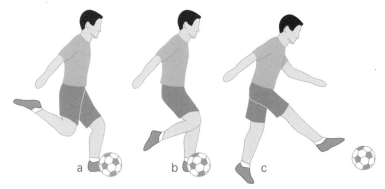

a   b   c

Movement of kicking leg/foot	Agonist	Antagonist	Plane	Axis	Type of contraction	Lever system
Hip action, flexion	Iliopsoas	Gluteus maximus	Sagittal	Transverse	Concentric	Third order
Knee action, extension	Rectus femoris (quadriceps)	Biceps femoris (hamstrings)	Sagittal	Transverse	Concentric	First order
Ankle action, plantarflexion	Gastrocnemius	Tibialis anterior	Sagittal	Transverse	Concentric	Second order

Hip, knee and ankle action in a jump

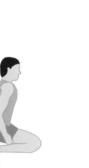

Movement upward phase	Agonist	Antagonist	Plane	Axis	Type of contraction	Lever system
Hip action, extension	Gluteus maximus	Iliopsoas	Sagittal	Transverse	Concentric	Third order
Knee action, extension	Rectus femoris (quadriceps)	Biceps femoris (hamstrings)	Sagittal	Transverse	Concentric	First order
Ankle action, plantarflexion	Gastrocnemius	Tibialis anterior	Sagittal	Transverse	Concentric	Second order

Hip, knee and ankle action in a squat

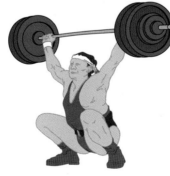

Movement downward phase	Agonist	Antagonist	Plane	Axis	Type of contraction	Lever system
Hip action, flexion	Gluteals	Iliopsoas	Sagittal	Transverse	Eccentric	Third order
Knee action, flexion	Rectus femoris (quadriceps)	Biceps femoris (hamstrings)	Sagittal	Transverse	Eccentric	Third order
Ankle action, dorsiflexion	Gastrocnemius	Tibialis anterior	Sagittal	Transverse	Eccentric	Second order

Practice makes perfect

1 Complete a movement analysis table for the hip, knee and ankle actions in the drive and recovery phases of running. *(1 mark per box)*

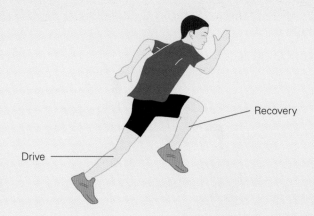

Drive

Recovery

(a) Drive

Joint	Movement	Agonist	Antagonist	Plane	Axis	Type of contraction	Lever system
Hip							
Knee							
Ankle							

(b) Recovery

Joint	Movement	Agonist	Antagonist	Plane	Axis	Type of contraction	Lever system
Hip							
Knee							
Ankle							

2 Name and sketch the lever system that operates at the ankle joint. *(3 marks)*

3 What do you understand by the terms mechanical advantage and mechanical disadvantage? *(4 marks)*

Chapter 7

Skill and ability

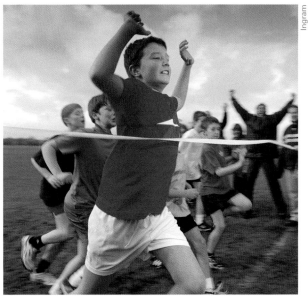

What you need to know

By the end of this chapter you should:
- know the difference between skill and ability
- know the characteristics and definitions of skill
- understand the difference between motor and perceptual abilities
- know the types of skill — cognitive, perceptual and psychomotor
- be able to develop a classification of skills according to distinct criteria

If you watch football on television, you will have heard the commentator remark on a particular player's great ability, especially when that player executes a skill in an effective way. The terms skill and ability are used frequently in sport, sometimes with confusion between the two, so we need to establish the differences between the two terms.

Ability

Abilities are the building blocks of skill. There is no such thing as general ability, but rather a group of abilities that are specific to a skill. For example, a sprint start in athletics requires the abilities of power, gross body coordination and speed. Abilities are therefore varied and numerous, and they combine in groups to be the foundation for the development of specific sporting skills.

> **Ability:** an innate characteristic that lays the foundation of skill.

Ability in sport is an innate characteristic required for performing movement. We might be born with good coordination, for example, which could help us to develop passing skills

Ability is evident from an early age

after periods of practice. We inherit natural abilities from our parents and while these abilities can be enhanced, the fact remains that you have either got it or you haven't!

Abilities are enduring. You born with them and they tend to remain with you. A player born with natural strength will retain that ability for life and be able to call upon it when required, especially if such natural strength is enhanced by weight training.

Examples of abilities include:

- explosive strength
- dynamic strength
- static balance
- dynamic balance
- speed
- power
- agility
- visual acuity

- gross body coordination
- manual dexterity
- stamina
- hand–eye coordination
- perceptual ability
- psychomotor ability
- gross motor ability

You are probably familiar with most of these abilities but some may be new to you. Visual acuity is the ability to scan the playing arena in order to pick up information. Manual dexterity is the ability to coordinate actions with the hands. The term dynamic refers to active movement, so dynamic balance is needed on the move, as in a gymnastic floor sequence, while static balance is needed during a handstand.

Perceptual ability is particularly important. It is the ability to sense and interpret information. For example, a netball player may have to assess how far away another player is before deciding how hard to project the ball when making a pass. Psychomotor ability is the ability to deal with information once you have sensed it. In other words, it involves the ability to make decisions based on information received. Having sensed how far away your team-mate is in netball, you might then decide on the best type of pass to use.

Gross motor ability is the characteristic required to perform large muscle-group movements, such as the strength needed to make a rugby tackle using the deltoid and latissimus dorsi muscles in the shoulder.

> **Key terms**
>
> **Perceptual ability:** the ability to sense and interpret information.
> **Psychomotor ability:** the ability to assess a stimulus and respond with the correct action.
> **Skill:** a learned, efficient movement performed with a purpose and to a consistently high standard.

Skill

Skill differs from ability in that it is not innate. Skill is learned, and developed from ability after a period of practice. To produce a skilled performance, the player must practise so that the underlying abilities are enhanced. Think of some skilful performances in sport, such as a magnificent free kick in football that bends around the defensive wall, or an exquisite performance on the ice by an Olympic skater.

Characteristics of a skilful performance

Skilled performances:

- are **learned**. On the basis of existing abilities, the practising of skills and drills in some form of training will help to produce a skilful movement.
- are **consistent**. A skilled player is able to perform the task to the same high level time after time. For example, a penalty taker in hockey might score nine penalty flicks out of ten during the season.
- are **goal-directed**. A player will practise skills with an aim in mind. He/she might want to improve shooting skills in order to score more goals.
- are **aesthetic**. They look good. A top-class dance routine is pleasing to watch.
- follow a **technical** model. A skilful performance will closely match a correct demonstration of the skill.
- are **controlled**. The skilful performer is in charge, controlling the rate and timing of the skill.
- are **efficient**. The skill is performed without any wasted energy.
- are **smooth**. The movement appears to flow.

The sports psychologist Knapp summed up the characteristics of skilful performance when he defined skill in sport as:

the learned ability to bring about predetermined results with maximum certainty, often with the minimum outlay of time, energy or both.

You should learn this definition since it includes many of the characteristics of skilful performance.

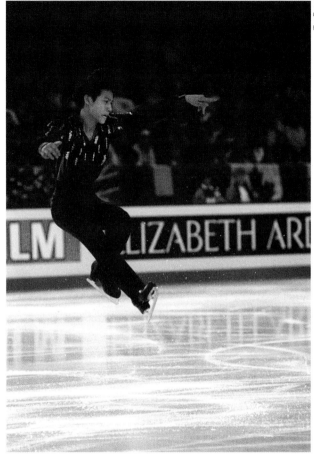

TopFoto

Skilful performers are great to watch!

Top tip

Exam questions often ask you to name three characteristics of skill. Make sure that you name three *different* characteristics because the examiner will mark the first three only. The terms goal-directed, consistent and learned would get the marks but the terms smooth, fluent and efficient might be considered too similar to gain separate marks.

Tasks to tackle 7.1

Draw a simple diagram or table to show a comparison of skill and ability.

A skilful performance has two elements:

- a **cognitive** part
- a **motor** part

The cognitive part of the skill requires thought before action. The motor part requires control and efficient movement. A football player about to make a pass must first look to see which other players are in a good position to receive the pass before the ball is kicked.

The relationship between skill and ability

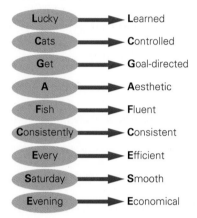

The following mnemonic might help you to remember the characteristics of skill for exam purposes:

Lucky	→ **L**earned
Cats	→ **C**ontrolled
Get	→ **G**oal-directed
A	→ **A**esthetic
Fish	→ **F**luent
Consistently	→ **C**onsistent
Every	→ **E**fficient
Saturday	→ **S**mooth
Evening	→ **E**conomical

The abilities we are born with are the foundations upon which skills are developed. However, abilities do not develop into skills overnight. The process by which abilities develop into skill is longer term and can be seen as a three-tier structure.

Abilities are innate. We are born with some of the abilities mentioned on p. 60 to varying degrees. These abilities can be enhanced during early years development by simple play or, even better, by good early coaching. Children who have access to good sports facilities and who are part of one of the many coaching schemes run by professional sports bodies are likely to enhance their natural abilities quickly. Children copy role models and are therefore more likely to pursue sports if they see their parents involved in sporting activities.

Abilities develop into fundamental or **foundation** skills. These include running, throwing, catching, kicking, balancing, jumping, hitting and evasion. They are the basic movements from which more advanced (**sport-specific**) skills develop. Sport-specific skills are learned after lengthy practice sessions and include such things as a javelin throw or a tennis serve. For example, a player born with the abilities of power, coordination and manual dexterity could enhance these abilities into the foundation skills of throwing and hitting, and these could in turn be developed into the sport-specific skill of the tennis serve.

The relationship between skill and ability is explained in Figure 7.1.

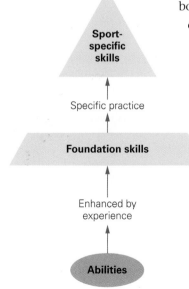

Figure 7.1 The skill–ability relationship

Skills classification

Skills classification can help sports practitioners to plan and prepare their coaching sessions. Skills are usually classified on a sliding scale called a **continuum**, which shows the extent to which a skill meets certain criteria. The continuum can also reveal how a skill varies depending on the situation. A continuum is a visual guide to indicate where a skill fits into a specific category. The criteria used to classify skills are detailed below.

Tasks to tackle 7.2

Name a skill from a sport of your choice and then name the abilities that underpin it and the fundamental skills from which it could have been developed. For example, a netball pass is built on the abilities of hand–eye coordination and manual dexterity, and developed from the fundamental skills of catching and throwing.

Environmental influence

An **open** skill is one that is affected by the sporting environment. The performer has to make decisions. Open skills are usually externally paced. Examples include a football pass, when the ball carrier has to decide which team-mate to pass to, or a tennis return that depends on the opponent's shot. In either case, the player has to adapt to the actions of others and make a decision on where to place the ball.

A **closed** skill involves less decision-making because it takes place in a more predictable environment and the performer knows exactly what he/she should be doing. An example is the shot put, which is always performed in a circle of the same size. The performer can use the same routine without much adaptation. A closed skill is self-paced: the rate at which it is executed is up to the performer. It can become a habit and tends not to be affected by the environment.

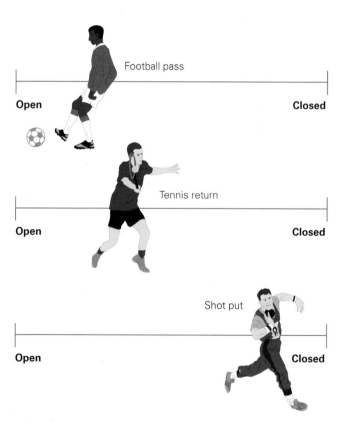

Figure 7.2 The environmental influence continuum

The environmental decisions continuum is shown in Figure 7.2. Note how the football pass and the tennis return are both open, but the football pass is more open than the tennis return. The continuum therefore shows the range between skills and, in the case of open or closed skills, by how much the coach needs to vary training so that a degree of adaptation is included in practice.

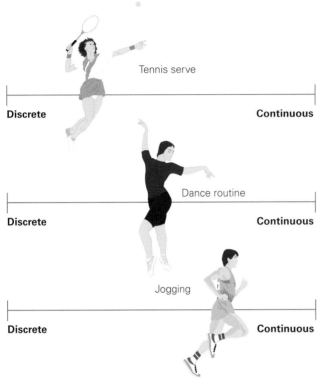

Figure 7.3 The continuity continuum

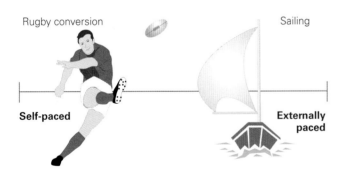

Figure 7.4 The pacing continuum

Continuity

A **discrete** skill has a short time span and a distinct beginning and end. An example is a tennis serve, where the action is short, sharp and clearly defined. A **continuous** skill has no clear beginning or end. The end of one part of the movement links into the next. An example is the leg movement in cycling or jogging. A **serial** skill is a set of discrete movements, linked together in a particular order to form a more continuous task. Serial skills therefore occupy the middle ground on a continuum, indicating that there are discrete elements that form a more continuous task. Examples include the leap, jump, turn and kick that might be linked together to form a dance routine, and the hop, step and jump that must be performed in a specific order in the triple jump in athletics. In both cases, each discrete movement can be practised separately.

Pacing

A **self-paced** skill is one during which the performer controls the rate of execution. The performer can decide how to execute the (usually closed) skill before doing so. Such pre-decision-making is called **pro-action**. For example, when a penalty is taken in football, the player can decide to place the ball in the corner of the goal or 'blast' it past the goalkeeper.

An **externally paced** skill is one during which the rate of execution is outside the control of the performer, who may have to react to external conditions. It is usually an open skill. In sailing, for instance, the speed of the wind dictates the pace of the boat, and the yachtsman or woman has to react accordingly. In an invasion game such as netball, the timing of the pass might depend on the pressure exerted by the opponents.

Muscular involvement

A **fine** skill has small, delicate muscle movements, such as the finger control required in a pistol shot at a target. A **gross** skill uses large muscle group movements, such as the movement of the biceps and triceps during a badminton drop shot. Most skills in sport are gross skills. A rugby tackle uses the deltoid muscle in the shoulder and is also a gross skill. The rugby tackle is further towards the gross end of the continuum than the badminton drop shot.

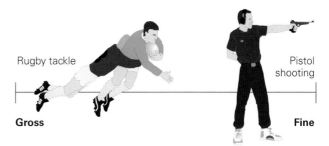

Figure 7.5 The muscle involvement continuum

Decision-making

A **complex** skill involves a high level of decision-making and has a large cognitive or thinking element to it. Examples include a passing sequence in netball or a set of tackles in rugby league. Players need to concentrate on the task and pay attention to numerous variables.

For a **simple** skill, such as a forward roll in gymnastics, the performer has a limited amount of information to process and the skill has a smaller cognitive element. The performer can concentrate on the task and focus on its successful completion.

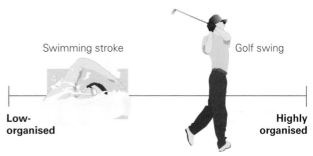

Figure 7.6 The decision-making continuum

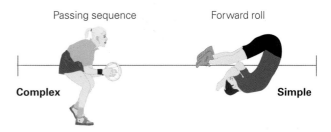

Figure 7.7 The organisation continuum

Organisation

A **low-organised** skill can be broken down into parts, or subroutines. The subroutines of the task can be identified as independent actions. For example, when teaching a swimming stroke, the arm and leg actions can be taught separately using a float. A **highly organised** skill is hard to break down since it is fast and ballistic in its execution. The parts that make up the task are integrated closely in the action. A golf swing is an example.

Tasks to tackle 7.3

Using the named skill from Tasks to tackle 7.2, classify the skill as open or closed, discrete, serial or continuous, externally paced or self-paced, gross or fine, complex or simple, and highly organised or low-organised. Give reasons for each classification.

When answering questions on skill classification be careful not to fall into the trap of describing the skill instead of explaining why it is classified as it is. For example, a football pass is open because it is influenced by the sporting environment and decisions are needed, not because the ball has to be kicked to another player and there are many players in a football team. Use a diagram of the skill classification continuum to show that you know the difference between types of skill, but make sure that you label it and name the skills to get the mark. It is a good idea to add notes to explain your diagram to make sure you are understood.

Practice makes perfect

1 Explain why there is no such thing as a general ability in sport.   *(2 marks)*

2 Explain why a continuum is needed to classify skills in sport.   *(2 marks)*

Chapter 8

Skill acquisition

Information processing

What you need to know

By the end of this chapter you should be able to:

- analyse the methods and processes by which information is collected from the sporting environment and coded
- explain how this information is stored in the memory
- explain the advantages of reacting quickly to information from the sporting environment

Ways to process information

In Chapter 7 it was noted that a skill can be divided into a cognitive part and a motor part. The cognitive part is concerned with thinking about and processing information before we use it. So information processing occurs in the initial stages of movement and looks at the ways that information is dealt with — an essential process before actions take place.

There are three stages to information processing:

- **Stimulus identification**. The player needs to pick out the important cues from the environment. For example, in cricket a fielder needs to pick out the flight and speed of the ball when the batsman hits it towards him before he can make a catch.
- **Response selection**. The second stage of information processing is decision-making. Once the stimulus has been identified, the performer must decide what to do with the information. The fielder has to decide how to make the catch — whether to move to the left or to the right and at what speed — based on the information he has gathered.
- The final stage is **response programming**. Having made a decision, the fielder has to instruct his muscles to make the required movement so that the action of making the catch can be performed. The brain sends a message to the muscles telling them to contract. The motor part of the skill can now take place.

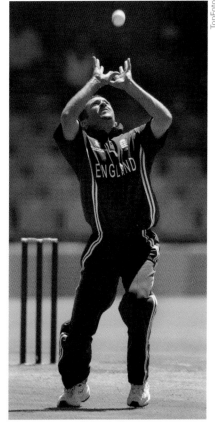

Howzat! Successful information processing brings rewards in sport

Information processing models

The mechanics of information processing in sport can be analysed in detail by reference to models. The models represent the mechanisms involved in the brain when information is dealt with as a flow chart — a logical sequence of events expressed visually. The two models available for study are the **Welford** and **Whiting** models (Figures 8.1 and 8.2).

> **Key term**
>
> **Information processing:** the methods used to deal with information collected by the senses.

Information processing terminology

The **display** is the sporting environment from which all information is gathered. It includes all the information available to the performer — whether relevant or irrelevant. For example, in tennis the display could include the essential items such as the ball and the position of the opponent as well as peripheral information such as the umpire and the crowd watching the game. At times the player might be tempted to pay attention to the crowd and not to hitting the ball, causing him/her to make errors.

Information is picked up from the display using the **senses**. All the senses are used in sport. For example, vision is used to track the flight of a ball

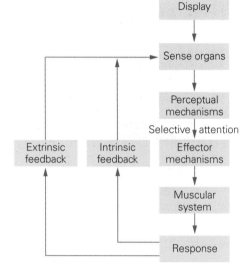

Figure 8.1 The Welford model

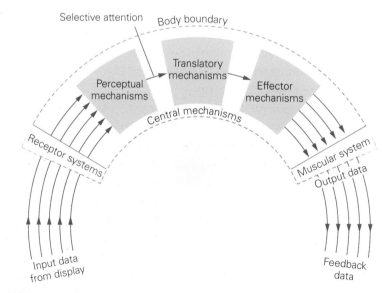

Figure 8.2 The Whiting model

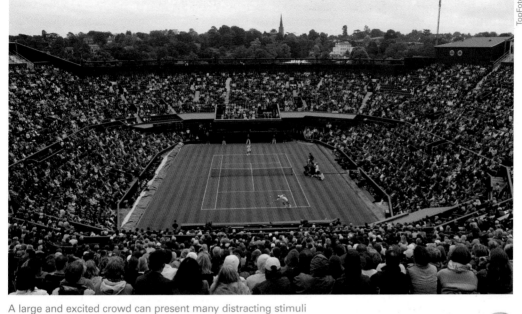

A large and excited crowd can present many distracting stimuli

Selective attention: **Key term** filtering of relevant information from irrelevant information.

and hearing or audition is used in team games — a player might hear the call of a team-mate, or pay attention to the referee's whistle. A sense of balance or equilibrium ensures that there is stability in the player before he/she makes a move. Balance is an essential requirement for gymnasts performing on the balance beam. Sports players are said to have a good sense of touch if they are able to weight a pass delicately into the path of a team-mate. The final sense used in sport is an inner sense. It tells the player how much tension is present in the muscles when they contract, and the angle at which the joints are placed. This inner sense is called **kinaesthesis** and it tells the athlete about body movements. A javelin thrower would know without looking that his/her arm is behind and held straight and high just prior to the release of the javelin.

With all the information present in sport and the variety of senses used to collect it, some sorting out is necessary to prevent the performer from becoming confused. Have you ever been trying to concentrate on watching a game on television, only to be disturbed by your brother or sister asking you a question? It is difficult to focus on two things at the same time, never mind a multitude of things. It is the same when you are playing. It is impossible to pay attention to *all* the information contained in the display without becoming confused and probably taking much too long to think about your next move. In the next stage of information processing — the **perceptual mechanisms** — the wealth of information picked up by the senses is filtered by **selective attention**. The relevant information is filtered from the irrelevant information so that the player is left with just the stimulus, or important information, to concentrate on. Irrelevant information (noise) is disregarded.

Once such relevant information has been filtered and **coded**, it is marked as important and any subsequent decisions can be based on the relevant information alone. **Decision-making** then takes place in the perceptual mechanisms. A right-handed tennis player, having determined that the ball is coming to the left-hand side, would decide to hit a backhand. In the Welford model, decision-making is included in the perceptual mechanisms but in the Whiting version it is given a separate identity — the **translatory mechanisms**. The Whiting model shows a reduced number of arrows going from the perceptual mechanisms to the trans-latory mechanisms, indicating that selective attention reduces the volume of information from the display, so that any decision is based on the stimulus alone.

When a decision has been made, it has to be communicated to the muscles so that movement can be initiated. The **effector mechanism** is the network of nerves that transport the decision from the brain to the muscles. In Whiting's model there are again several arrows going from the effector mechanism to the muscles, indicating that more than one set of muscles are used. These muscles are triggered into action by the effector mechanism. It is now possible for **muscular contractions** to take place. These muscular contractions facilitate movement so that the motor part of the skill, the actual **response**, can take place.

The performer can be helped by **feedback** — information given after the response to promote movement correction. Two types of feedback are shown in Welford's model. **Intrinsic** feedback comes from within the player, who might know when he/she has over-hit a shot. **Extrinsic** feedback is given by the coach.

Tasks to tackle 8.1

1 What do you understand by the terms **display** and **selective attention**?

2 What types of feedback would you use for a beginner in sport?

Top tip

Information processing involves definitions and specific terminology that you must be familiar with. Learn all these new terms off by heart. You might be asked to explain what you understand by any of the features of the information processing models, so make sure you know them all and that you can define each feature and illustrate it with an example.

Memory

Once information has been processed, it can be stored so that it can be used again in similar sporting situations. The memory system stores and codes the results of the information processing mechanisms. It consists of a number of stores and ways of moving information between the stores. The **short-term sensory store** is a temporary storage facility. It works quickly, taking only a fraction of second to hold and code all the information from the sporting environment. The information from the display is collected using the senses and then almost immediately this wealth of information is filtered using the process of **selective attention**. It is necessary to filter the information from the display to avoid information overload.

The relevant information or stimulus is sent to the **short-term memory**. This has a limited capacity and can only deal with about seven items of information at any one time. The short-term memory is often called the working memory because it has many functions. It receives the relevant information from the sensory store and uses this information to initiate movement. It then passes this information to the **long-term memory**. Information can remain in the short-term memory for about 30 seconds before it is either lost or moved to the long-term memory.

Once the information has been logged into the long-term memory, it remains there for a long time. The long-term memory has an unlimited capacity and can store a lifetime of information. When you were of primary school age you may have learned how to ride a bike. Even if you did not ride your bike much at secondary school, you will not have forgotten how to. The information is stored in the long-term memory in the form of a motor programme — a method of storing the components of a task in a logical sequence.

There is a two-way relationship between the short-term memory and the long-term memory. They work in tandem so that information can be moved from the short-term to the long-term memory for storage and then retrieved at an appropriate time in the future.

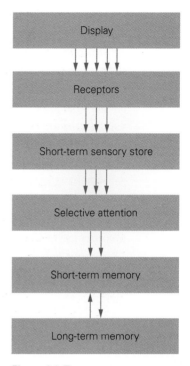

Figure 8.3 The memory system

Coding information in the long-term memory

It is important for the coach to be aware of the two-way relationship between the long-term and the short-term memory systems, so that movement patterns can be stored in the long-term memory and used by the performer when needed. The coach can enhance the process of storing motor programmes in the long-term memory by making the player practise the task repeatedly. During such practice the coach should offer praise and reinforcement to the player, because we tend to remember pleasant experiences. We also tend to remember unpleasant experiences. For instance, if you are injured making a bad tackle, you will remember it. For the same reason, the coach might use punishment to emphasise what not to do.

Skills are more likely to be remembered if they are associated with other items already stored in the memory. If you are trying to learn an overarm volleyball serve and you already know how to serve in tennis, the coach might let you start by thinking about the tennis serve.

People can often recall where they were and what they were doing when some major event took place. If the coach makes sessions unusual in some way, the learner will recall the information by associating the session with the learned task. Coaching sessions should be fun and enjoyable.

Mental rehearsal involves going over the task in your mind. It stimulates the brain and the associated muscles and so helps to store information in the long-term memory. The coach should ensure that demonstrations are clear and accurate, so that players do not recall inaccurate information.

Information can be stored in the memory more easily if it is broken down into small pieces, so that the relevant information can be focused on. This process is called **chunking**. When giving feedback or advice to the player, the coach should present the information in small, relevant parts, rather than giving all the information at once.

If this information follows a sequence, or chain, then the coach should link the information given to the player, starting with the first part of the task, the grip of the ball for example, before going on to present information about the subsequent passing movement. This process of **chaining** will help to preserve the task in the memory in the correct order.

> **Tasks to tackle 8.2**
>
> List the features of the short-term memory and the long-term memory.

Motor programme theory

Imagine that you are an experienced athlete and that you have been practising the skill of a shot put for many years. When you compete at a major event, the performance of the shot put is the same as it has been during all those years of practice, because it is a closed skill and is not affected much by changes in the environment. Your movements are controlled by a motor programme.

> **Key term**
>
> **Motor programme:** a set of movements, stored in the long-term memory, that specify the components of a task or skill.

A motor programme is a set of movements, stored in the long-term memory, that specify the components of a skill. A motor programme is formed by specific and continued practice. As a skill is practised, images are built up in the long-term memory and the effective actions are stored while the incorrect and negative aspects of performance are eliminated. Internal and external feedback help to check errors and amend performance continually. The net result is the storage of a perfect image that can be called upon for future use.

The use of a motor programme to control movements has obvious advantages. The player, having perfected the task with practice, is in the autonomous phase of learning and therefore has almost automatic control of movement. The performer is able to concentrate on the finer aspects of the task and pay attention to detail. Movements are smooth and efficient and reaction times are quick. An expert basketball player is able to score from a free throw at the edge of the key after a foul because he/she has practised this skill many times.

Motor programmes are stored in the long-term memory to be retrieved when required. They are stored in the form of an image that contains both the required task (sometimes called the executive) and the subroutines that make up the executive. For example, the skill of a tennis serve is made up of the subroutines of the grip, the ball placement, the throwing action, the trunk rotation and the arm action.

Motor programmes can be developed from an early age by practice. Such basic motor programmes become the foundation for more complex motor programmes at a later stage. In Chapter 7 we noted how foundation skills such as throwing are developed by early practice. The motor programmes for these foundation skills might become an essential part of a more complex task, such as a tennis serve, which uses the ball toss (a throwing action) as an essential subroutine.

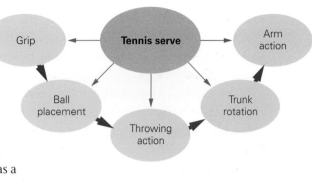

Figure 8.4 Tennis serve motor programme

The problem with motor programmes is that they cannot be used for open skills because the movement will need to be adjusted according to changes in the environment.

Reaction, movement and response

It is a great advantage to the athlete if information collected and stored in the memory can be dealt with quickly. It takes only fractions of a second to go through all the mechanisms required to process information but if those mechanisms can be speeded up even more, then that extra fraction of time enables the performer to read the situation and gives a little more time to select the appropriate action.

Before reacting to a stimulus the performer needs to:
- receive information from the display via the senses
- code this information into relevant and irrelevant items using selective attention
- make a decision based on the relevant information — select the response
- initiate the response by sending impulses to the muscles

In relative terms, coding the information and making a decision take longer than receiving the information and initiating the response but all four activities take place just prior to actual movement. Therefore **reaction time** involves no movement. It is the time taken from the

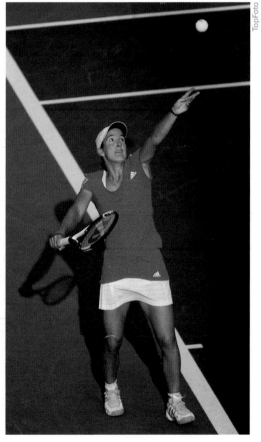

A tennis serve is made up of a series of subroutines

presentation of the stimulus to the onset of the movement. **Movement time** is the time it takes to complete the task from start to finish. The **response time** is the time taken from the presentation of the stimulus to the completion of the task — it is the sum of the reaction time and the movement time. Figure 8.5 shows the relationship between response time, reaction time and movement time.

In the 100 metres sprint, the reaction time is the time from hearing the gun to the point just before leaving the blocks. Movement time is the time from leaving the blocks to hitting the tape at the finishing line. The response time is the time from hearing the gun to hitting the tape.

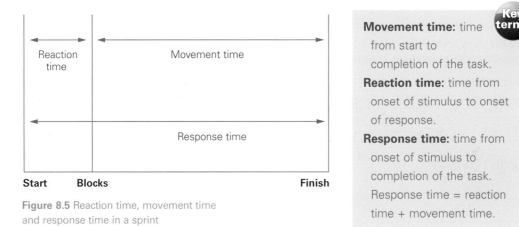

Figure 8.5 Reaction time, movement time and response time in a sprint

> **Key terms**
>
> **Movement time:** time from start to completion of the task.
> **Reaction time:** time from onset of stimulus to onset of response.
> **Response time:** time from onset of stimulus to completion of the task. Response time = reaction time + movement time.

Influences on reaction time

The time it takes to react, and therefore to respond, to a stimulus is influenced by a number of factors.

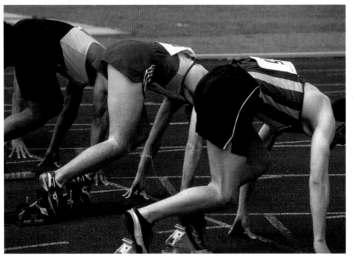

Colin Underhill/Alamy

A quick reaction is vital for success in sprinting

The number of stimuli

The more choices available, the slower the reaction will be. A simple reaction time can be very fast because it involves only one choice to one stimulus. For example, the only response of an athlete to hearing the starting gun is to push away from the blocks and run as fast as possible. A choice reaction time involves more decision making and usually takes more time. For example, a midfield hockey player must choose which player to pass to from a number of available team-mates. However, the relationship between reaction time and the number of choices is not linear. The *rate of* increase in reaction time decreases with increasing choice. Hicks's law describes the relationship between the number of choices and reaction time (Figure 8.6).

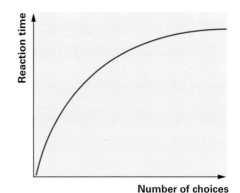

Figure 8.6 Hicks's law

Hicks's law states that, although having more choices makes performance slower, the rate of increase in reaction time decreases as the number of choices increases. For example, a goalkeeper faced with two attackers who are clean through on goal might rush out and pressure the player with the ball. This increases the ball carrier's choices. He has to go around the goalkeeper, pass to his team-mate or shoot, and making the decision will cause him to hesitate. On the other hand, footballers are told by the coach not to dive in at the feet of an opponent with the ball in midfield but rather to hold their position and see what the attacking player does before making a move. This is because the attacking player already has a number of options to choose from and adding one more will increase reaction time only by a small amount, according to Hicks's law.

Experience

A player's experience will affect the reaction time. Experienced players can anticipate the bounce of a ball and get there first. Have you ever played squash against a more experienced player? You might have found yourself chasing the ball around the court while your wily opponent always seemed to be in the middle of the court exactly where the ball landed. Anticipation, or the ability to pre-judge a stimulus, is a major influence on reaction time.

The ability to anticipate comes with experience. Guessing what your opponent is going to do is easier if you can get a feel for the way the pitch or court is playing. For example, tennis players need to get a feel of the court if they are changing from the clay courts of the French Open championships in Paris to the grass courts of Wimbledon. This process is called **effector anticipation**. Anticipation can also be improved by gaining prior knowledge of the opponents from your coach, or by watching the opponents before you play them. This prior knowledge is called **perceptual anticipation**. Players can also gain information on their opponents during the game by looking at the way they shape up to make a play, the stance or the grip on the ball. Picking up such cues from the environment is called **receptor anticipation**. Whichever method is used to aid anticipation, the performer should remember that it is a gamble. If you anticipate correctly, reaction times and response times will be reduced and there will be more time to play your shots and concentrate on detailed aspects of the performance. You will also suffer less from fatigue. However, if your gamble is wrong and you make the wrong guess, reaction times and response times will increase dramatically and you may not have time to make the play.

Gender and age

Studies have shown that men tend to react faster than women but women retain their ability to react quickly until much later in life. Ageing slows the reactions of both men and women.

Performance-enhancing drugs

Performance-enhancing drugs can affect reaction time. The infamous start made by Ben Johnson in the 100 metres at the 1988 Seoul Olympics was made under the influence of performance-enhancing steroids.

Stimulus intensity

The intensity of the stimulus can affect reaction time. Athletes tend to react faster to a stimulus that is loud or bright, such as the loud bleep at the start of a swimming race, or the brightly coloured cricket ball that is played with during night matches.

Fitness

Reaction times will be quicker if the player has trained to improve his/her physical fitness.

Improving reaction time

Two theoretical concepts that explain reaction time are the single-channel hypothesis and the psychological refractory period.

The **single-channel hypothesis** suggests that a stimulus is processed along a single nerve track and that the brain can only process one stimulus at a time — think about the capillary network, which allows only a single blood cell to pass through at any one time. The single-channel hypothesis implies that any subsequent stimulus must wait for the one before it to be processed before it can be dealt with, rather like a queue of cars waiting at a road junction. The single-channel hypothesis is illustrated in Figure 8.7.

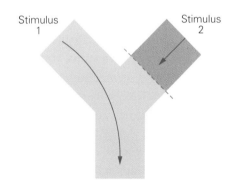

Figure 8.7 The single-channel hypothesis

The **psychological refractory period** is based on the single-channel hypothesis. It too suggests that only one stimulus can be processed at a time, and if a second stimulus is presented to the performer before the original one is processed, then an unavoidable delay will occur. This delay is known as the psychological refractory period (PRP). The PRP occurs because the second stimulus must wait for the first one to be processed, even though the first stimulus is no longer valid. An example of this phenomenon is the ball hitting the net in tennis and deflecting in a different direction from which it was originally travelling. A dummy pass in rugby is an attempt to present a first stimulus to the opponent, who begins to follow the flight of the imaginary pass. When the player keeps the ball and runs with it, the opponent is momentarily confused and the reaction is delayed. Experienced players often use the PRP to their advantage by using dummies or body language to present two stimuli to their opponents in quick succession, so that there is no time to deal with the first stimulus before the second is presented.

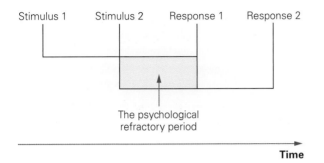

Figure 8.8 The psychological refractory period

Exam questions often ask for definitions of reaction time, movement time and response time. Reaction time is an important feature of performance, so make sure you are able to suggest ways in which a coach can improve the reaction times of players.

Practice makes perfect

1 How could a sports coach ensure that information is stored in the long-term memory of a sports performer? *(4 marks)*

2 Define the terms **reaction time**, **movement time** and **response time** in terms of sport. *(3 marks)*

What you need to know

By the end of this chapter you should:
- know the three phases that performers pass through as they develop their skills
- be able to present practical examples to show how a coach could help a player to progress from the early to the latter stages of learning
- understand the theoretical concepts that explain how learning sports skills can be achieved

The phases of learning

The psychologists Fitts and Posner proposed that learners pass through three stages as their skills develop. These three stages are known as the phases of learning.

The cognitive phase

This is the first phase of learning experienced by a beginner who tries to work out and understand what is required to perform a new movement. The novice might watch a demonstration of a skill and then try to perform the task with uncoordinated movements. It is a short phase during which a trial-and-error process is used to help develop an early understanding of the parts of the skill. The performer in this phase uses closed-loop control and relies heavily on feedback. Time is needed to think and to check movements. The coach might use manual and mechanical guidance and concentrate on extrinsic and positive feedback to offer encouragement and ensure improvement.

> **Key term**
>
> **Closed-loop control:** at lower levels of performance, feedback is used to control actions. Such feedback, available after the response, is used to help control the next movement, implying a continuous or closed-loop mechanism.

The associative phase

This is often called the practice phase of learning. The learner compares his/her current level of performance with that of a top-level player. Long periods of practice and the use of feedback to correct errors are needed to perfect the skill. Trial and error may again be used to achieve a smoother performance and fine-tune any errors. The feedback during the trial-and-error process may be internal, from within the player, who may now have more idea of the perfect movement. During this phase the player begins to build up a mental framework of the task, with the parts of the skill — its subroutines — coded in the memory. This framework is called a **motor programme**. The performer should now be able to use intrinsic feedback and begin to alter the level of skill, using negative feedback. Verbal and visual guidance could be used.

The autonomous phase

This is the third and final phase of learning. At this stage movements are perfected to the point where they are almost automatic. The player can concentrate on the finer details of the task and the performance is completed with maximum efficiency. A football player at this level can do a pass almost without thinking about it and can now perfect that pass by weighting it to perfection. This is a phase for experts, who must continue to practise if they want to remain at this top

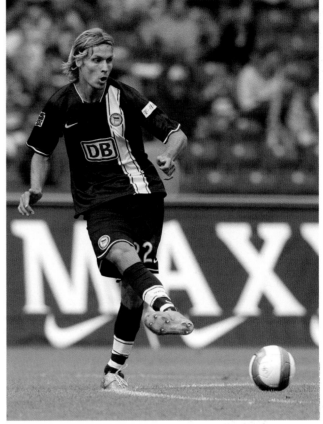

Professional footballers can pass quickly and with little thought

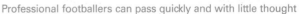

level. Motor programmes are firmly stored in the memory. At this high level of performance the player could benefit from both intrinsic feedback and from advice from the coach (extrinsic feedback). Any guidance is tactical and verbal.

Coaches can use strategies to help players to progress from the early cognitive phase to the final autonomous phase of learning. An understanding of some of the theoretical concepts behind these strategies will further enhance learning. Learning leads to a permanent change in behaviour and movement patterns. However, performance is a temporary response to a situation and can still fluctuate. The psychologist Steve Bull summed it up as follows:

> Learning may be considered to be a more or less permanent change in performance associated with experiences [while] performance may be thought of as a temporary occurrence fluctuating from time to time due to many operating variables.

Top tip

Exam questions often refer to the three phases of learning. Make sure that you know a couple of salient points about the cognitive, associative and autonomous phases, backed up by examples so that you can describe the key characteristics of each phase.

Tasks to tackle 9.1

Suggest what types of practice, feedback and guidance you might use for performers in the cognitive phase, the associative phase and the autonomous phase of learning. Information on practice and guidance can be found on pp. 166–172. Information on feedback can be found on pp. 173–174.

Motivation

Motivation is defined as the external influences and internal mechanisms that arouse and direct our behaviour. This implies that motivation is a powerful tool that can be used to shape the behaviour of an athlete. Motivation affects the amount of effort that a player puts into the game and players with a strong will to win are usually more successful. Players who are motivated will persist with the task, even when the odds are against them. A team that is a goal down with only a few minutes left to play will benefit from players who are well motivated, because they will keep trying until the end of the game to score a last-minute goal.

Motivation also affects performance relative to ability. A coach might motivate novice performers by offering rewards and incentives, such as a 'player of the week' award. A beginner who feels he/she is doing well in an activity will increase in confidence and want to continue to improve.

More experienced players may be motivated by their own success. The knowledge that they have had a good game is enough. The motivation will still be there for the next game.

This more permanent type of motivation is called **intrinsic motivation**. Intrinsic motivation comes from within the performer and is characterised by feelings of pride and satisfaction from completing or succeeding in a task. A feeling of enjoyment may be derived both during and when reflecting on the performance. Examples of intrinsic motivation include the thrill of scoring a goal, the satisfaction of winning a major competition and the pride you feel on reaching the top of a mountain after a difficult walk. The feeling of well-being derived from such motivation ensures that the performer maintains the desire to continue with the activity and hence intrinsic motivation is long lasting.

Extrinsic motivation is more temporary. It includes both tangible and intangible rewards from an outside source. Intangible rewards are non-physical, such as the praise and encouragement given by the coach to a beginner who has performed well on the early part of a task, or to a championship athlete after a record-breaking performance. There may not be a trophy but the applause from the crowd brings satisfaction. Tangible rewards include the medals and trophies that are awarded to players at the end of the season, or for player of the match. Other examples include the certificates given to young swimmers as they progress through the early swimming grades, or the money on offer to professional players when they sign a new contract.

Both extrinsic and intrinsic methods of motivation can be used to help sports performers of all grades, but the coach should use these two types of motivation carefully and appropriately. Extrinsic rewards are a good way of attracting newcomers to an activity, and young performers in particular are delighted to receive certificates or medals for any early success that they achieve. However, although extrinsic rewards may provide the foundation for future participation, they should not be used all the time. The continued use of praise and rewards may mean that a player participates for the 'trophy', rather than for the pleasure of taking part. In this way the overuse of extrinsic motivation may undermine intrinsic motivation. The coach should offer praise and reinforcement whenever possible, especially to beginners, but remember to limit the use of extrinsic rewards as the player gains experience.

Intrinsic motivation is desirable because it is a more permanent way of maintaining interest in an activity. The coach should gradually decrease the extrinsic rewards and replace them with intrinsic motivators. Setting personal goals for the performer and then giving ownership of those goals to the performer can promote intrinsic motivation.

Other ways for a coach to motivate players include making training sessions fun. A variety of activities and some 5- or 6-a-side games could be introduced. The coach could also adjust the training environment to suit the players — for example, small groups may be planned so that players of similar ability train together. The coach could inspire players by pointing out role models. These need not be established star players but should include players of good ability, perhaps from within the club, who are well respected. The achievements of such lesser role models can appear to be within reach of novice players rather than being impossible to achieve.

As players gain experience, more demanding goals can be set. An athlete who has reached a personal best should be praised for the achievement and then set another higher target to meet. The coach should stress that goals achieved are due to the ability and effort of the player. In other words, success should be attributed to internal factors. Personal improvements can be emphasised as a reason for individual or team success. The coach should

ensure that tasks set at the start of a training programme are within the capabilities of the performer. By allowing success, the coach provides confidence and a desire to continue training.

The greatest benefits from motivation can be gained by rewarding specific behaviour. An improvement in a particular technique that has been worked on in recent weeks could be praised. It could be emphasised that a better performance is a direct result of the improvement.

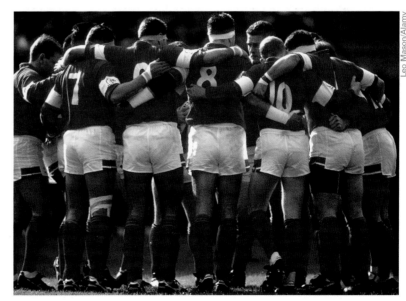

Motivation before a match

The coach should consider the personality of the performer before deciding on the best way to offer motivation. Extrovert individuals enjoy the limelight and can be praised openly. Others might prefer to be praised quietly, away from other people. Motivational praise should be given as soon as possible after a performance. A young player receiving the player of the match award at the team meeting immediately after the game will feel proud.

The learning curve

When a novice is learning a new closed skill, he/she passes through four stages that can be represented on a graph (Figure 9.1).

At stage 1 the novice is working out the subroutines of the task and performance is at a low level. The performer is in the cognitive phase of learning and the performance may appear uncoordinated.

At stage 2 there is a rapid increase in the rate of learning as the performer begins to master the task. The performance is more fluent and executed with enthusiasm. The success achieved provides reinforcement and motivation.

At stage 3 the performer hits a plateau and there is little or no improvement in performance. The plateau effect could be a consequence of the performer reaching the limit of his/her ability, or becoming bored with performing the same task.

At stage 4 there is a reduction in the level of performance, possibly due to fatigue or loss of motivation. The initial drive to succeed has been lost, a concept called **drive reduction**. A new challenge or extension to the task is needed to maintain motivation.

To avoid the plateau and dip in performance at stages 3 and 4, a coach should provide rewards and encouragement to maintain motivation. The plateau concept should be explained to the performer so that he/she understands the slow down in improvement. The performer may be given a break to offset fatigue.

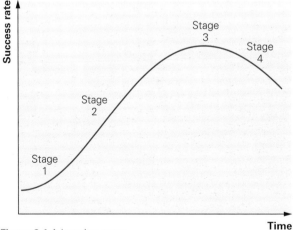

Figure 9.1 A learning curve

A learning curve is a graphic illustration of how a performer's rate of learning a closed skill can vary over a period of time. The initial stage that involves working out the required subroutines of the task can be quite brief, perhaps a few hours, but the performer may remain in stage 2 for some weeks as performance improves.

The cognitive theory of learning

The cognitive theory of learning suggests that we learn by working out the solutions to problems ourselves.

A performer learns by thinking about and understanding what is required, rather than simply developing a series of responses to various stimuli. The problem is solved as a whole, using previous knowledge and experience. For example, an athlete in a long-distance race may work out that the best way to beat the other runners who have a faster finish is to set off at a fast pace. If this tactic works, the performer might be motivated to repeat the same response when confronted by a similar problem in the future.

To work out solutions to problems, the performer must develop an understanding of the tactics required. Past experiences may be used to find the correct response. The solution to the problem (referred to in cognitive theory as an **intervening variable**) is arrived at because the athlete understands why he/she is choosing a particular course of action.

Gestalt (from German 'pattern', 'form' theory) supports the cognitive theory of learning by suggesting that problems are best solved using a whole approach, rather than focusing on just part of the task.

> **Key term**
>
> **Cognitive theory of learning:** learning based on solving problems using past experience and concentrating on the whole skill.

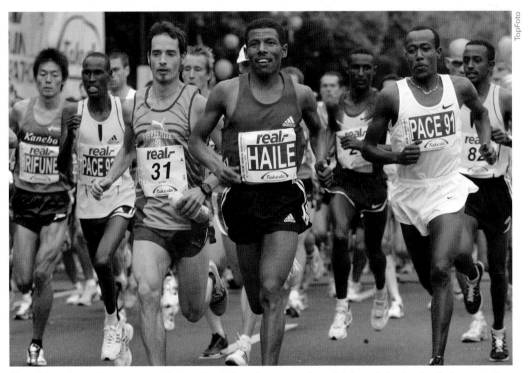

Elite athletes know their opponents' strengths and weaknesses and use this knowledge to plan their race tactics

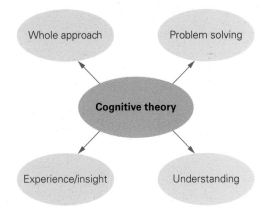

Figure 9.2 The cognitive theory of learning

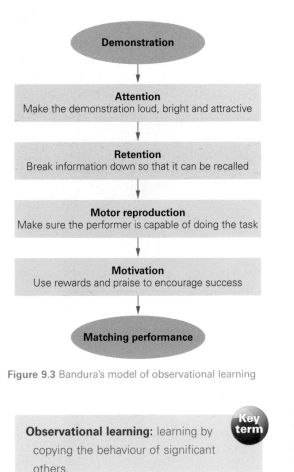

Figure 9.3 Bandura's model of observational learning

Observational learning: learning by copying the behaviour of significant others.

Key term

Make sure that you differentiate between the cognitive phase of learning and the cognitive theory of learning. Under the pressure of an exam, it is easy to misinterpret a question and write about the wrong topic.

Top tip

Tasks to tackle 9.2

Give a practical example for each of the four elements of cognitive theory displayed in Figure 9.2.

The observational theory of learning

When children are playing football in the park, they often celebrate scoring a goal by pulling their shirts off and running around the pitch. They are copying the behaviour of the professional players they have seen on television. Sports coaches can use the fact that significant behaviour is often copied by using strategies to ensure that the learner copies desired behaviours.

The psychologist Bandura suggested that behaviour and demonstrations are more likely to be copied if they are consistent, so it is important to give accurate demonstrations each time. Behaviour is more likely to be repeated if it is re-inforced with success, particularly if it is a powerful image performed by a role model. Bandura suggested that there are four principles that should be followed (Figure 9.3).

Attention

The learner must be attracted to the demonstration. The coach should grab the player's attention by making the image powerful, bright and relevant. Cues should be used to highlight key points.

The coach is responsible for 'selling' the skill to the performer by pointing out its function. For example, it could be suggested that the reason for learning a new pass in rugby is to allow the ball to be transferred faster to create more time to beat the defence. Reference to an effective pass by a top player might add to the attractiveness of the task.

Retention

Once the player has accepted the idea of a new skill, the coach must make sure that it is remembered. The information should be broken down into bite-size pieces so that it can be processed more easily in the short-term memory, which has a limited capacity. Practice and repetition must take place to ensure that the skill is learned thoroughly.

Motor reproduction

The performer must have the ability to do the task. During early learning the coach should demonstrate basic skills. For example, the basic grip on the ball in rugby must be correct before a pass is attempted. The coach should make sure that the player has the necessary coordination and power in the arms and shoulders to make the pass.

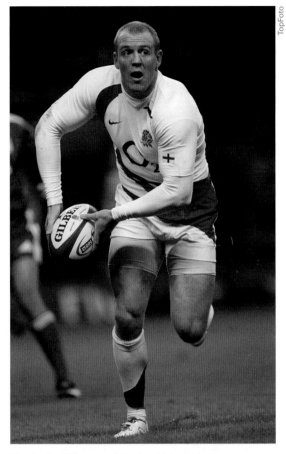

The basic skills are required at all levels

Motivation

The learner is more likely to continue to practise and learn if he/she is motivated. The coach can motivate players by offering positive reinforcement in the form of praise or rewards when the demonstrated skill is copied correctly. Most sports governing bodies have award schemes for young players who can successfully demonstrate specific skills.

Transfer of training

The theory of transfer explains that the learning and performance of one skill can be affected by the learning and performance of another.

There are six types of transfer. An understanding of the different types of transfer can be useful to both the coach and the player.

Proactive transfer is when a skill learned previously is used to help one being currently developed. For example, a netball player might use

Key term

Transfer of training: the effect of the learning and performance of one skill on the learning and performance of another.

a netball pass to help in the initial stages of playing basketball. She is using a skill she already has to affect the performance of a new task. **Retroactive transfer** is when a skill being learned currently interferes with a skill already learned. When the netball player returns to netball training after playing basketball, there may be some effect on her netball pass.

In **positive transfer** the learning of one skill is aided by the learning of another because of similarities in execution. The skills must have a similar shape and form, so they are built on similar abilities. For example, a tennis player might be able to use the subroutines of the tennis serve to help in learning an overarm volleyball serve. Both tasks involve a throwing action, an overhead hit and a trunk rotation, and the subroutines of both tasks are used in a similar way. As the performer develops, feedback could be used to refine the task so that the volleyball serve becomes more technically correct.

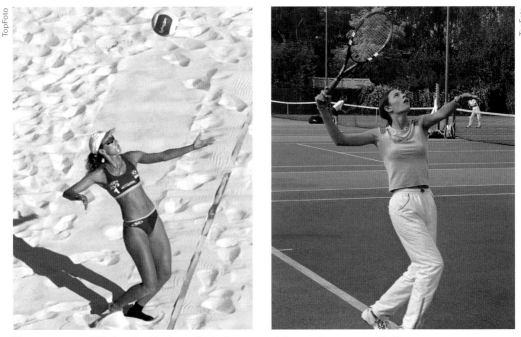

The movement skills involved in the volleyball serve and the tennis serve are similar

Negative transfer also occurs in the initial stages of learning, but in this case the learning and performance of one skill is hindered by the learning and performance of another. Negative transfer occurs when two tasks have some similarities but are not identical. A strike in rounders and a cricket shot both involve striking actions but a rounders ball is hit one-handed and at waist height. If you attempted a cricket shot in this way you would most likely be bowled out. The subroutines of the tasks are used in different ways.

Negative transfer is an unwelcome phenomenon for sports performers but with a little specific practice and some help from the coach it can be resolved. Remember that the effects of transfer occur in the initial stages of learning. Negative transfer may occur because the player fails to understand the requirements of the task, or because he/she tries to use a skill from one game in a different and inappropriate environment. The coach should point out the specific requirements of the task.

Zero transfer is often confused with negative transfer. For negative transfer to occur there must be some resemblance between the two tasks. In zero transfer there is no such similarity and therefore there are no effects of the learning and performance of one skill on another. Two skills such as swimming and rock climbing are so different that there is no learning effect from one to the other.

In **bilateral transfer** a learned skill is transferred from limb to limb across the body. A good coach will always encourage players to use both sides of the body. A right-handed basketball player needs to be able to do a lay-up shot with either hand. A left-footed football player needs to practise with the right foot, and a rugby player who is better at passing from the right hand should try passing from the left hand.

Positive transfer is most beneficial and there are ways that a coach can encourage it. Simply pointing out the concept of transfer to a player might help. One of the best ways to promote positive transfer is to offer a realistic approach to training and practice. For example, in the early stages of learning to dribble in hockey, the coach may use cones (and no defenders) to make it easy to master the task. In the later stages of learning, the players have to transfer this skill to the real game. The coach should therefore introduce opponents in practice sessions and perhaps do drills that involve the attack against the defence to simulate a real game situation. The more realistic the practice, the more beneficial it is likely to be.

One way to use the concept of positive transfer during training sessions is to make sure that the tasks are performed in a progressive manner, so that the easiest part of the skill is well learned before moving on to a more difficult aspect of the task. For example, when learning a pass, a performer might concentrate on the grip of the ball before progressing to the actual passing technique and then to passing against passive opponents.

The coach can use positive reinforcement to make the most of positive transfer. When a player brings a skill from a previous game and uses that skill to good effect, the coach might praise the player and say, 'We can use that to start with and build on it.'

Schema theory

Schema theory is similar to transfer of training. The sports psychologist Schmidt suggested that the theory of transfer can be enhanced by using the ideas or concepts of the task that form the basis of the skill. Schema theory suggests that the same skills can be used in different sports because the performer has developed a general set of concepts that allows skills to be adapted to suit the situation.

Top tip

Exam questions on the theories of learning require detailed revision. An exam question will typically ask you to say what is meant by a key point and then ask you to apply your understanding of that topic. For example, you might be asked what positive transfer means and how you would ensure that positive transfer occurs.

Top tip

Make sure you know the difference between positive and negative transfer and appropriate examples to show the difference between them.

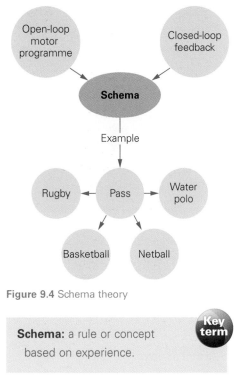

Figure 9.4 Schema theory

Key term

Schema: a rule or concept based on experience.

A schema is therefore a rule based on experience. A motor programme that has been developed for a well-learned skill such as a netball pass could be adapted using feedback so that the pass could be used in basketball. There are similar principles behind the execution of a pass in both games. They both involve passing to a target player, they both involve grip of the ball and both require an arm action and a follow-through.

To initiate a pass in either game the player could use the basic concepts of passing stored in the memory in the form of a motor programme and adapt them with some internal feedback to suit a particular situation. In other words, the principles of passing stored in the memory could be used for a basketball or a netball pass. Further experience could allow the pass to be used in rugby or even water polo so that, rather than a concrete, well-defined skill, the performer has a set of concepts available to suit the situation (Figure 9.4).

A schema is general in the sense that it can be used in different sports, but it is also specific. Passing, for example, is a particular skill.

Feedback is an essential feature of developing a schema because its use in adapting the existing motor programme is important.

The schema is developed in four parts:

- The **initial conditions**. In the first instance the player needs to gather information from the environment, such as the position of other players. For example, a basketball player making a pass needs to take in information from the environment to determine his/her own position on court as well as the position of team-mates.
- The **response specifications**. The basketball player now needs to decide what to do. As a result of an awareness of the initial conditions, the player can decide on the best type of pass to use, to which player and how far the ball needs to be projected.
- The **sensory consequences**. The player gathers sensory information to help adjust the weighting and timing of the pass. He/she uses vision to sense the best available recipient of the ball. The sense of touch helps gain a feel for the pass.
- The **response outcome**. When the pass has been delivered, the player might receive information on the outcome. Did the pass reach its intended target?

The first two parts of the schema — the initial conditions and the response specifications — initiate the action and are called the **recall schema**. An experienced player will have faced similar situations before and can recall a plan or outline of the skill from memory.

The third and fourth parts of the schema — the sensory consequences and the response outcome — are called the **recognition schema**. They require the performer to use sensory information to adapt the task, using feedback gained from the environment. The recognition part of the schema is responsible for controlling the movement.

Schema theory is a useful learning tool for the coach and player. The coach should encourage the development of schemata by expanding the player's experience with a variety of practice and using positive reinforcement when the player uses a schema successfully. Most coaches vary their training sessions for team games, so that, for example, the attack might play against the defence in a variety of situations. Such variety is the best way to build a schema. If a particular player does well on a task, praise and encouragement should be offered.

> **Top tip**
>
> The four parts of schema theory should be learned well so that you can recall them should you be asked.

Operant conditioning and the stimulus–response bond

> **Key terms**
>
> **Operant conditioning:** shaping the environment to manipulate behaviour.
>
> **S–R bond:** the link between the stimulus and the response.

The S–R bond is the link between a stimulus and a response. In sport we learn by associating the correct response with a stimulus. For example, in badminton if an opponent hits the shuttlecock high and short to the middle of the court, the appropriate response is a smash shot. It is an advantage to the badminton player to learn to recognise when the smash is the best course of action and the coach can help to promote such recognition by using the right approach in training. The theory of operant conditioning explains how correct responses to a stimulus can be made stronger if the action is reinforced and the coach manipulates the performer during and after the performance.

Skinner studied rats in captivity. The rats quickly learned to hit a lever which presented them with food. Skinner called this process of learning to repeat actions for reward **operant conditioning**. Skinner's work showed that we learn by trial and error. If the response is correct then we are motivated to repeat it. If the response is incorrect we should be motivated to change it. For example, a tennis player who hits the first serve into the net will lift the ball higher on the second serve.

Operant conditioning works on the principle that actions are made stronger by repetition. When correct actions are reinforced, a stronger link to the stimulus is developed. Incorrect actions that are not reinforced make a weaker link to the stimulus.

A coach can accelerate the trial-and-error learning process by using strategies to:

- make the adoption of the correct response stronger
- make the neglect of the incorrect response stronger

The tactics used to demote the significance of the incorrect response are as important as the promotion of the correct response.

The strategies used to strengthen the S–R bond and promote adoption of the correct response are as follows:

- Use **positive reinforcement**. This is defined as something that increases the likelihood of the correct response being repeated. Positive reinforcement involves giving something pleasant after the correct response, such as praise and rewards.
- Allow **early success**. The coach should set easy targets at first to ensure success. A marker or a target could be drawn on the court for a player learning to serve in tennis to help get the ball on the right spot. If the player finds the serve difficult, he/she should be allowed to move in towards the net. Initial success develops confidence in the player and offers an incentive to continue.
- Use **mental rehearsal**. Going over the performance in the mind helps to develop an automatic response to the stimulus.
- Practise the **task as a whole**. The coach should allow the performer to practise the skill in its entirety as soon as he/she is able, in order to promote fluency and understanding of how all the subroutines come together.

Incorrect actions can be weakened so that they are eliminated. The coach should do the following:

Top tip

Learn the difference between positive and negative reinforcement. Positive reinforcement is adding a pleasant stimulus such as praise when you get it right and negative reinforcement is taking away that praise when you get it wrong.

- Use **negative reinforcement**. If the performer begins to make mistakes, the coach withdraws the praise and encouragement that he/she has been giving for doing the task well. For example, a swimming coach might stop praising a swimmer who has been doing a nice leg action when the leg kick begins to deteriorate with fatigue. The idea is that the swimmer will be motivated to apply more effort in order to regain the praise and encouragement from the coach.
- Use **punishment** when actions are incorrect. Coaches should use punishment carefully to avoid lowering the player's confidence while at the same time trying to prevent repetition of the unwanted response. Forms of punishment include being fined, booked, penalised, dropped from the team or made to do extra training.

Negative reinforcement is often confused with punishment. Negative reinforcement is best remembered as taking something (the incentive) away.

Thorndike suggested three laws to link the stimulus to the response and promote learning:

- The **law of exercise** states that practice will strengthen the S–R bond. Players who practise regularly quickly recognise the appropriate response to a stimulus. Repetition of skills and drills in training sessions can produce movements that are almost automatic responses to the stimulus.
- The **law of effect** states that a satisfier such as praise will strengthen correct responses and that an annoyer such as criticism will weaken incorrect actions. Encouragement and praise

are good ways to motivate and generate the drive to keep producing the correct response. Players do not take kindly to criticism and will be motivated to prevent negative comments from the coach by changing incorrect actions.

- The **law of readiness** states that any task set by the coach should be within the capabilities of the player. The task should be challenging so that a sense of achievement is fostered. The performer must be both mentally and physically prepared to do the task. For example, a swimming coach would not expect a beginner to swim long distances or in the deep end. Simple drills in the shallow end would be practised to start with.

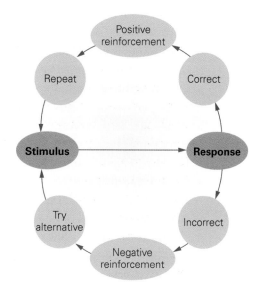

Figure 9.5 Learning by trial and error

Goal setting

Studies into sports psychology have found a positive link between goal setting and improved performance. Players who set targets for themselves, or have goals set by their coach, generally produce better results because goals provide specific boundaries and give the player something to aim for. This gives personal motivation and a sense of satisfaction when the target is reached. Goal setting also has an important role in lowering anxiety and reducing the stress of performing at high level.

The goals set by coaches and players can be long term or short term (Figure 9.6). Long-term goals are concerned with the end result of a lengthy period of work and are sometimes called **outcome** goals. A swimmer aiming to qualify for regional team selection before next year's championship is an example. Short-term goals are the stepping-stones to meeting long-term targets. Short-term goals can be performance-related, or judged against a past performance. An attempt by a swimmer to beat her personal best time by the end of next month is a step towards meeting the regional target time. Short-term goals can also be process-related or

> **Top tip**
>
> Learn Thorndike's laws for making the S–R bond stronger.

Tasks to tackle 9.3

List the differences between positive and negative reinforcement.

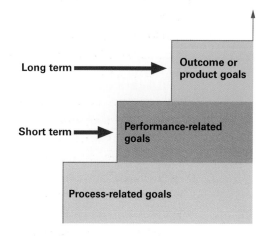

Figure 9.6 Stepping stones to success

concerned with technique, so in order to achieve a personal best time the swimmer must work on improving her exit from a turn.

It is important that goals do not focus solely on winning. In an athletics race, for example, there can be only one winner and performers who fail to reach their goal of winning might lose motivation and suffer stress. Coaches should set personal targets for individuals to improve performance and technique. Personal goals provide intrinsic motivation and may lead to longer-term success. You might not win the race but you can still gain a personal best time and show improved technique.

The SMARTER principle sets out guidelines for a coach to follow when setting goals:

- Goals should be **specific** and detailed. For example, instead of telling a performer to improve fitness, the coach should tell him to go up one level on the bleep test.
- Goals should be **measured** using statistics or a stopwatch so that both coach and player can see if they are making progress.
- Goals should be **agreed** between coach and player so that the player has ownership of the goal-setting process and feels more motivated.
- Goals should be **realistic** — they should be challenging but achievable.
- A **time scale** should be set so that the difference between short-term and long-term goals can be identified.
- Goals should be **exciting** so that the player is engaged and motivated.
- Goals should be **recorded**, so that progress can be evaluated.

There are a lot of technical terms associated with the theories of learning. It would be a good idea to make a check list as you revise to make sure you know them all.

Practice makes perfect

1 One way to ensure that learning takes place is to develop the link between the stimulus and the response. How can a PE teacher ensure that a player chooses the correct response to a stimulus? *(4 marks)*

2 Transfer of training is the effect of the learning and performance of one skill on the learning and performance of another. Use examples from sport to explain any **two** types of transfer of training. *(4 marks)*

Chapter 10

Characteristics and objectives of physical activity

What you need to know

By the end of this chapter you should be able to:

- understand the characteristics and objectives of the concepts of play, physical education, leisure and recreation, active leisure, outdoor and adventurous activities (OAA) and sport
- compare and contrast these concepts with one another
- illustrate the benefits of play, physical education, active leisure, outdoor and adventurous activities and sport to individuals and to society in general

Leisure time

Characteristics

Leisure can be defined as spare time during which individuals can choose what to do. As a hard-working PE student, your leisure time may be limited because there are a lot of things you *have* to do, such as going to school or college, earning money through a part-time job, doing your homework or coursework and so on. When all your duties have been completed, you might have a little time left to spend as you wish. This is your leisure time and you can spend it in various ways, such as going to the gym, or playing the latest computer game. Many people like to relax and spend their leisure time inactively. Others look for excitement and danger — it is a matter of **personal choice**.

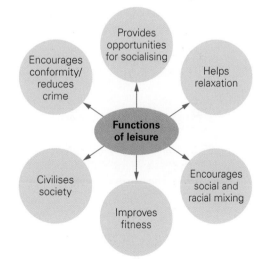

Figure 10.1 Functions of leisure

Objectives

When used positively, leisure serves many purposes both for individuals and for society in general (Figure 10.1). For individuals, leisure helps people to **relax** and **unwind**, gives them the opportunity

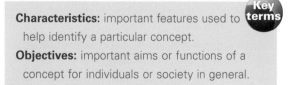

Characteristics: important features used to help identify a particular concept.
Objectives: important aims or functions of a concept for individuals or society in general.

Key terms

to **socialise** and meet other people, and allows for improvements in **health** and **fitness**. They can develop physical skills and improve their confidence and achieve a sense of self-fulfilment.

For society in general, leisure can encourage **conformity**, **civilise society** and encourage **social and racial mixing**.

It is sometimes difficult to separate individual from social functions of leisure as they often overlap. For example, individual improvements in health and fitness reduce the demands on the NHS for society.

The term 'leisure' covers a variety of types of active participation, for example play, physical recreation and sport. Physical education is a compulsory subject at school and as such lessons cannot be considered leisure time. However, school PE programmes can 'educate for leisure' and provide extra-curricular options for pupils in their free time.

Tasks to tackle 10.1

Do the following examples fit the description of leisure time (yes or no)?
(a) watching sport on television
(b) going to a pub quiz with friends
(c) doing your homework
(d) playing football professionally
(e) going to school or college for AS PE lessons

If you were asked, 'What are the objectives of physical education?', 'development of skills' is too vague an answer to earn any marks. It is important to state clearly the type of skills being developed, e.g. physical skills, social skills, cognitive skills.

Figure 10.2 illustrates an activity continuum containing different concepts that vary in relation to features such as degree of organisation, structure etc.

Low structure	High structure
Non-competitive	Highly competitive
Choice	Obligated
Spontaneous	Organised

Play	Physical recreation	Outdoor recreation	PE	OAA	Sport

Figure 10.2 The leisure continuum

Factors influencing leisure-time activities

A number of factors can affect a person's participation in active leisure (Figure 10.3). These include:

- **socioeconomic status** — i.e. how much time and disposable income someone has
- **stereotyping** — traditional viewpoints may limit participation in leisure-time activities that 'go against the norm', for example female bodybuilding and male dancing

- **disability** — local facilities and availability of specialist coaches are often inadequate for accommodating people with disabilities
- **age** — some activities are seen as being suitable only for the young, for example skateboarding
- **ethnicity** — some ethnic groups do not place as high a priority on 'active leisure' as they do on educational achievement and religious observances
- **lack of facilities** — while people may have plenty of free time, local facilities are often limited or of poor quality

Barriers to participation are explored in more detail in the section on equal opportunities on pp. 140–46.

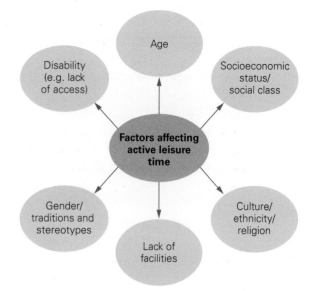

Figure 10.3 Factors affecting active leisure time

It is important to be able to both list and explain the factors influencing how we spend our leisure time. For example, for people with disabilities, access is a key issue in getting to and around facilities.

Leisure time is not always spent actively. Some people choose to spend it sedentarily (inactively), for example reading, watching television or listening to music. Active leisure time includes a wide range of activities, for example hill walking, swimming and playing netball.

Physical recreation

Characteristics

Recreation can be defined as the **active** aspect of leisure. It is entered into **voluntarily** during **free time** and people have a **choice** concerning which activities they take part in. The focus is on **participation** rather than results.

A number of key features help to identify physical recreation. It is **flexible** in relation to rules, time spent on an activity and space used. The atmosphere tends to be **relaxed** — taking part is the main motive. For example, an adult having fun with friends while taking part in a relatively energetic physical activity is engaged in physical recreation.

Recreation can be identified by its emphasis on participation, as opposed to competitiveness, which is linked more to sport.

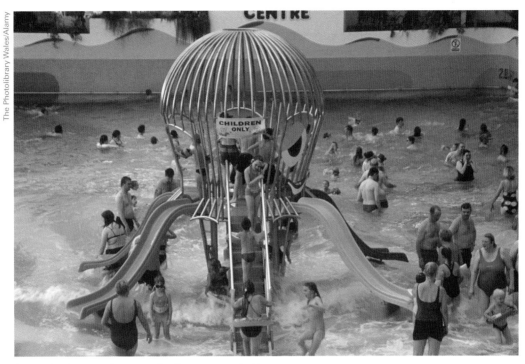

Swimming is a popular recreation for young and old

Objectives

Recreation provides many benefits, including the opportunity to:

- relax and unwind
- socialise and meet new people
- be creative and do something you are proud of (self-fulfilment)
- improve health and fitness

Such benefits explain why recreation is important to individuals in our society.

Almost everyone has the opportunity to take part in some kind of recreation. Venues can be chosen and agreed by participants who decide when to take part (i.e. what time of day) and how regularly.

A key reason why many people take part in recreational activities is to relax and recuperate from the stresses of everyday life, for example work and family responsibilities. Playing team

Top tip

Questions often require an understanding of the benefits of recreation and active leisure for individuals or society in general, and these often overlap.

Tasks to tackle 10.2

Consider the following examples of people taking part in physical recreation:

(a) a group of workmates playing five-a-side football every Thursday night after work

(b) a group of teenagers training regularly to improve fitness at a boxing club after school

List the benefits that individuals and society would receive from such participation.

games helps them to gain social benefits as well as improve fitness. Outdoor pursuit activities may encourage creativity. Achievement of personal goals helps to develop self-esteem.

Recreation can also be said to increase conformity and morality in society as a whole. Social benefits of recreation include:

- community integration through mass participation events
- less strain on the NHS
- social control and crime reduction
- employment opportunities
- economic benefits

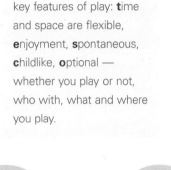

The mnemonic '**tesco**' is useful for remembering some of the key features of play: **t**ime and space are flexible, **e**njoyment, **s**pontaneous, **c**hildlike, **o**ptional — whether you play or not, who with, what and where you play.

Play

Characteristics

When physical activity is identified as 'play', it generally has to be:

- fun — designed for enjoyment and non-serious
- spontaneous — a spur of the moment decision to play
- simple and childlike in nature
- non-rigid — rules and time and space boundaries should be flexible
- self-administered — participants determine the rules and time for play

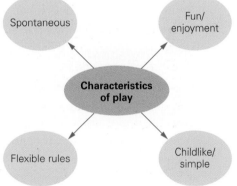

Figure 10.4 Characteristics of play

Equipment may be modified and simple, often using what children bring with them, for example jumpers used as goalposts.

If you observe children participating actively in a fun, enjoyable manner, with little or no adult interference, then you have a number of key characteristics that identify the activity as play.

For example, children and adults (*who?*) can take part in swimming in a playful manner in a paddling pool at the local park, or in a pool at a leisure centre (*where?*). *When?* is decided by the participants, often on the spur of the moment. Most take part to have fun (*why?*), splashing about in the water in a non-serious manner (*how?*).

Comparing and contrasting play and recreation

Characteristics shared by play and recreation include the following:

- They are entered into of one's own free will.
- The primary motivation is enjoyment.
- They have an informal structure — for example, flexible rules and time.
- The outcome is non-serious, and a casual attitude is adopted.

Differences between play and recreation include the following:

- While intrinsic motivation is the primary aim for both play and recreation, other motives are likely to be involved in the recreation process — adults may use recreation to escape the stresses of daily life, and view it as an opportunity to improve their health and well-being.
- While both play and recreation have a flexible, loose organisation or structure, recreation is slightly more organised than play.

It is important that you are able to identify shared characteristics of concepts, as well showing your knowledge of differences between them.

Objectives of play

Play has many different functions both for adults and children.

The key feature of adult play is **motive**. For an adult, play has mainly psychological benefits as it can provide stress relief, an escape from the reality of everyday life, recuperation from daily duties and an opportunity to relax. This is important in the modern-day lives of many individuals as they have stressful jobs with long working hours. There are often many demands on time and money, which can cause stress. Reverting to childhood and engaging in activity in a playful manner can serve as an important stress release.

The main function of play for a child is to master reality. It gives the opportunity to discover what it is to take on an 'acceptable role' in society. Through play, children learn many things including:

Make sure you can distinguish between the key values of play for a child (mastering reality, learning about life) as opposed to those for an adult (escape from reality, relaxation).

- social skills, such as making friends and cooperation
- physical skills, such as coordination
- emotional skills, such as accepting defeat
- environmental skills, such as safety awareness
- cognitive skills, such as decision making
- moral skills, such as fair play

Sport

Characteristics

Sport can be defined as a contrived competitive experience and is identified by a number of key features. It is **goal-orientated** and involves **competitiveness** (i.e. the will to win). It is **serious**, particularly at the elite level. **National**

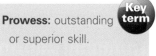

Prowess: outstanding or superior skill.

governing bodies look after the interests of, and try to develop the popularity of, particular sports. They also provide strict **rule structures** that are enforced in **competitions** by officials. Sport requires high levels of **physical skill (prowess)** and **effort** (endeavour) in order to succeed and gain the **extrinsic rewards**, such as trophies or money, that are on offer.

An element of **chance** is often involved in sport and can mean the difference between winning and losing. **Time and space restrictions** apply and **specialist equipment** may be required. A high level of **commitment** to training is needed to improve performance and fitness.

The levels of seriousness, commitment and skill in sporting involvement vary. Some individuals are talented enough to take part professionally (i.e. they earn their living from sport). Others participate in sport as amateurs during their leisure time at a local netball, hockey or cricket club for example.

Sport is therefore different from recreation in that it is competitive, strict rules apply and extrinsic rewards are available.

Key characteristics of sport
Serious/competitive — 'win at all costs' attitude or sportsmanship (*how?*)
Prowess — high skill levels, particularly by 'professionals' (*who?*)
Organised — sport has rules/regulations (*how?*)
Rewards — available for winning (extrinsic) and intrinsic satisfaction (*why?*)
Time and space restrictions apply (*when?/where?*)

Figure 10.5 Key characteristics of sport

Table 10.1 A comparison of physical recreation and high-level sport

Physical recreation	High-level sport
Immediate pleasure	Sometimes enjoyable, particularly in victory, but may involve anxiety and pain
Participation provides intrinsic rewards and enjoyment	There may be extrinsic rewards
Length of participation is the individual's own choice	Time constraints on training or length of game
Spontaneity exists	Less spontaneous because of game plans
Level of training is the individual's own choice	Serious training is required
Flexible rules	Strict rules

The more you can identify features such as competition, high skill levels and physical exertion, the more likely it is that the activity can be classified as sport.

Make sure you can compare sport and recreation.

Functions of sport

Sport serves a number of important functions for individuals including:

- improved health and fitness
- increased self-esteem and self-confidence
- opportunities for socialising

Participation in sport also has a number of important benefits for society. Some of these are similar to the benefits of recreation, including less strain on the NHS as people's health and fitness increase, and improved social control as people's free time is spent in a positive manner. Sport can help to integrate society through participation by different socioeconomic or ethnic minority groups. The sporting success of national teams creates national pride, for example England becoming rugby union world champions in 2003 and winning the Ashes in cricket in 2005. Economically, sport provides financial and employment benefits. For example, money is invested into provision of sports facilities, and sport provides jobs and regeneration opportunities, as illustrated by the London Olympics for 2012.

Tasks to tackle 10.3

How many marks would you award the following answer?

Q Identify four characteristics of sport. *(4 marks)*

A ● improved fitness
 ● increased social control
 ● improved integration in society
 ● more jobs on offer in society

$-$ $+$

Gamesmanship	Sportsmanship

Examples of gamesmanship	**Examples of sportsmanship**
– Playing on despite injury to opponent	+ Kicking the ball out if an opponent is injured
– 'Sledging' — using verbal insults to put an opponent off and affect his/her performance	+ Verbally congratulating the positive performance of an opponent
– Diving intentionally to try to gain a penalty	+ Trying to stay on your feet and score despite a late tackle

Figure 10.6 The gamesmanship–sportsmanship continuum

Sporting ethics

When participating in sport, performers adopt various codes of behaviour, which can be viewed on a continuum. At one end is **sportsmanship**, which involves treating the opponent with respect and as an equal, fair play and playing within the rules or etiquette of the game. At the other end is **gamesmanship**, that is, the use of unfair practices to gain an advantage, often against the etiquette of the game, but sometimes without actually breaking the letter of the law, for example wasting time at the end of a game when you are winning.

Such codes of conduct can have positive or negative effects on the sporting contest. On the one hand, sportsmanship can help a game to run smoothly and encourage goodwill among players and spectators. On the other hand, gamesmanship can lead to ill feeling and a contest disintegrating as officials struggle to make decisions and keep control. Anger among players and spectators lowers the status of sport and leads to negative role models.

Gamesmanship is evident in modern-day professional sports, such as football, and has filtered down to amateur and school sports performers who copy the negative behaviour of their role models.

Physical education

Physical education (PE) can be defined as a formally planned and taught curriculum, designed to increase knowledge and values through physical activity and experience. Soon after becoming prime minister in July 2007, Gordon Brown stated his desire for all pupils to experience 5 hours per week of PE at school, including competitive school sports.

PE serves a number of functions (*why* do we teach PE?) that justify its existence as a National Curriculum subject. These include:

● developing **physical skills**, for example coordination, body awareness
● developing **social skills**, for example communication, cooperation, forming friendships

- developing **mental** or **cognitive skills**, for example decision-making, self-control
- improving **health** and **fitness** through activity and knowledge of the benefits of exercise
- developing **self-esteem** and confidence through **success**
- developing **leadership** skills
- helping to prepare young adults for **active leisure** when they leave school, for example via school–club links and taster sessions at local sports centres

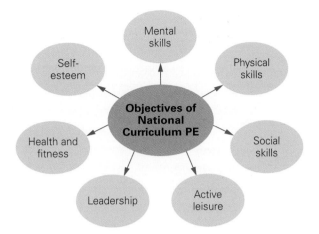

Figure 10.7 Objectives of National Curriculum PE

PE is delivered mainly to children and young adults (*who* is taught?), in schools and colleges (*where* PE is delivered). It is delivered mainly in lessons, at lunchtimes or after school (*when* PE is experienced) by teachers using a variety of teaching styles and activities (*how* PE is delivered).

Tasks to tackle 10.4

List and explain four functions of PE as a compulsory National Curriculum subject for children from age 5 to 16.

A triangular model of PE

A pupil's experiences of PE should involve three elements:
- education
- sport
- recreation

Education

Pupils experience National Curriculum PE from the age of 5 to age 16 as a compulsory subject. They are taught a range of activities and physical skills in a number of different areas of activity:
- games
- athletics
- swimming
- gymnastics
- dance
- outdoor and adventurous activities
- exercise activities

A number of different roles should be experienced, including performer, coach and official. The development of PE as a National Curriculum subject is explored in more detail on pp. 120–124.

Sport

Sport gives pupils an opportunity to experience organised, optional, extra-curricular activities with a competitive element. They might be chosen to play for the school netball team or to compete in an inter-schools swimming gala.

Recreation

Pupils can choose to engage in non-competitive physical activity in extra-curricular time. Many schools and colleges have open-access clubs for this purpose.

These three elements can be combined in a single lesson. For example, during a swimming lesson a coach may instruct pupils about technique (education), a race may be held (sport) and free time may be given at the end of a lesson when the pupils are allowed to choose what they want to do (recreation).

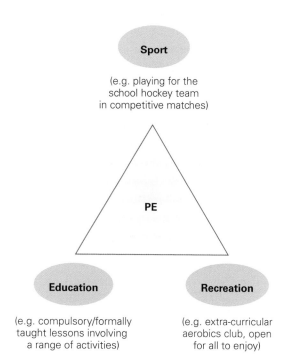

Figure 10.8 A triangular model of PE

Outdoor and adventurous activities

Outdoor and adventurous activities as education

Outdoor and adventurous activities (OAA) form one of the six areas of National Curriculum PE. OAA can be defined as 'the achievement of educational objectives via guided and direct experiences in the natural environment'. For example, pupils who are up a mountain and being formally instructed in skills such as map reading and taking a compass bearing are taking part in OAA.

Functions of OAA in the National Curriculum

OAA have many purposes, including raising awareness of and respect for others, oneself, the natural environment and danger or risk. Risks should be perceived only (i.e. in a pupil's head) rather than real (actual danger).

Outdoor activities such as hill walking, caving and canoeing can give personal

Top tip

Outdoor activities need to be specifically linked to the natural environment, for example mountain walking and rock climbing. Such activities as part of compulsory National Curriculum PE belong under the overall umbrella of PE, and so involve the same potential set of values (physical skills, health and fitness improvement, and social and cognitive development).

challenges to individuals, as well as teaching them how to work effectively with each other (teamwork, cooperation). They can provide opportunities to experience the responsibilities of leadership, such as making decisions that affect the rest of the group. Communication skills and an awareness of an individual's strengths and weaknesses may develop.

A sense of adventure and excitement is an important element of the outdoor experience.

Despite its compulsory status as part of National Curriculum PE, OAA in most schools tends to be of relatively low quality. A number of factors may negatively affect a pupil's OAA experience.

- If staff are lacking in specialist qualifications, experience or motivation, the opportunities for a positive and meaningful experience will be reduced.

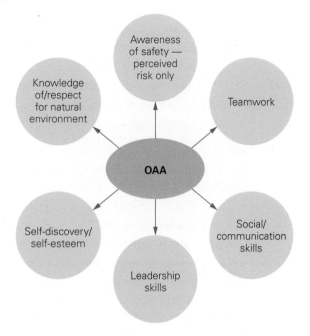

Figure 10.9 Functions of OAA

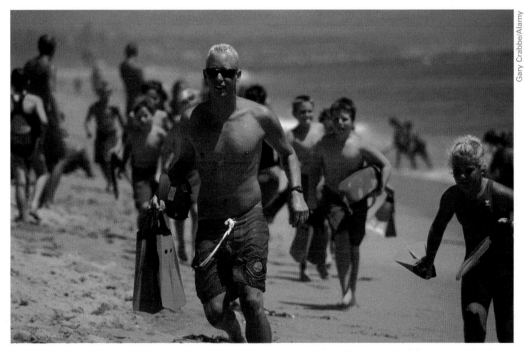

Staff in charge of OAA need to be well qualified and experienced in order to provide a meaningful and safe experience for students

- Lessons do not allow much time for such activities.
- Access or transport to the natural environment is a problem for many schools.
- Money and resources — the expense of undertaking OAA may be too much for many schools and parents. Specialist equipment may not be readily available.
- Parents and teachers are likely to be deterred by the inherent risks of certain activities such as skiing and mountain climbing. Negative media publicity of injuries to children participating in these activities has fuelled existing concerns.

It is the element of risk, danger and unpredictability that distinguishes outdoor education from the rest of the PE experience. Teachers should ensure that the natural environment that pupils experience is as predictable as possible, that is, under the control of the participant and not open to unpredictability such as flash floods and rock falls.

Top tip

It is important to be able to give a critical evaluation of a pupil's OAA experience in relation to the factors identified above, and to appreciate that in many schools it is taught in a limited manner due to such issues, for example orienteering activities may be restricted to the school grounds.

Outdoor and adventurous activities as recreation

The key characteristics and functions of physical recreation are defined and explained on pp. 95–97. The key distinguishing feature of outdoor recreation is that it takes place in the natural environment, for example climbing a mountain or canoeing down a fast-flowing river. The challenge of the natural environment is therefore a key identifying feature of OAA as outdoor recreation. Freedom of choice in leisure time distinguishes outdoor recreation from OAA as compulsory National Curriculum PE.

Tasks to tackle 10.5

Consider the following activities. If they could fulfil the characteristics of OAA as part of National Curriculum PE, explain how. If not, give reasons why.
- cycling
- hockey
- running

Functions of OAA as outdoor recreation

Individuals who choose to participate in outdoor recreational activities such as skiing and rock climbing do so for a number of reasons including:
- to improve health and fitness
- for stress release and relaxation
- as a personal challenge, to develop self-esteem and self-confidence
- to develop an appreciation of the natural environment

- to develop cognitive skills and decision-making
- to develop social skills and work as a team
- to develop survival skills

Reasons for increased participation

Nowadays, most people have more free time and disposable income. There has been continued interest in spending this free time and money pursuing outdoor recreational activities such as canoeing and rock climbing. Reasons for choosing outdoor recreation as leisure time activities include:

> **Task to tackle 10.6**
>
> Using an example, explain how an outdoor adventurous activity could be classified as sport.

- the positive portrayal by the media — snow boarding and mountain biking, for example, are seen as 'cool'
- an increased desire for excitement — the adrenaline rush
- participation is non-competitive, which makes them a good alternative to traditional competitive sports such as football and hockey

Practice makes perfect

1 Identify four key characteristics of sport. *(4 marks)*

2 Define the term **outdoor recreation**. *(2 marks)*

3 Modern-day lifestyles are becoming more stressful and less active. Explain the term **active leisure** and explain why it is important for individuals and society. *(4 marks)*

4 Young children often engage in play activities. State the benefits of play for young children. *(4 marks)*

5 List three educational values of outdoor and adventurous activities. *(3 marks)*

Facility provision

What you need to know

By the end of this chapter you should be able to:
- understand the key characteristics and goals of the public, private and voluntary sector provision for active leisure
- understand the advantages and disadvantages of such provision by the different sectors
- explain the concept of 'best value' in relation to public sector provision for active leisure

There are three main sectors you need to know about in relation to active leisure provision in the UK. Your need to know the key characteristics and aims of:
- the public sector
- the private sector
- the voluntary sector

Public sector

Public-sector organisations are owned by local authorities and trade on a profit-and-loss basis. Leisure provision includes leisure centres, swimming pools and skateboard parks. Key aims for public-sector organisations are high-quality recreational services and the promotion of mass participation in sport. The public sector has a number of important features that separate it from the private and voluntary sectors.
- Facilities are open to all — they are non-exclusive.
- They are run by local authorities and managed by local authority employees.
- They are run as business operations, with the aim of breaking even.
- They trade on set prices according to pre-set budgets.
- The facilities and services are of adequate or improving standard.

Aims of public-sector provision

Central government sees active-leisure provision as being increasingly important in modern society because of health and obesity issues. By providing facilities and schemes to increase participation in physical activity, local authorities aim to:

Public-sector provision: active-leisure opportunities provided by local authorities. Examples include public parks and leisure centres.

- increase health and fitness of individuals and improve the health and well-being of the community
- increase social control and reduce crime in the community
- improve social integration
- provide for social needs, equal opportunities and social inclusion
- regenerate areas (this may link to national government policy)

Such aims need to be achieved within financial constraints — it is a requirement to break even and to give taxpayers value for money.

Private sector

Private-sector organisations are privately owned businesses that promote activities to make a profit. In order to attract 'clients', the facilities and services offered have to be of a very high standard. Fitness clubs such as Fitness First and the David Lloyd health clubs are examples of private-sector organisations.

Characteristics of private-sector active leisure provision include:
- exclusive, selective clientele — elitist
- privately owned or registered companies
- trade on profit-and-loss accounts — the main aim is to make a profit
- managed by owners or appointed employees
- offer a high-quality service and facilities (at a price)

Membership of private fitness clubs has become increasingly attractive to the general public in our health-conscious society. Advantages of private-sector clubs are that individuals have more choice of where to go to improve their health and fitness, with such clubs offering high-quality facilities and service to encourage continued participation.

> **Key terms**
>
> **Private sector:** business operations offering active leisure opportunities with the ultimate aim of making a profit.
>
> **Social inclusion:** active leisure can help individuals who have little going for them (for example, no job, poor housing, no educational qualifications) to feel part of society, rather than feeling excluded.

> **Tasks to tackle 11.1**
>
> List three examples of public-sector active-leisure facilities in the area in which you live.

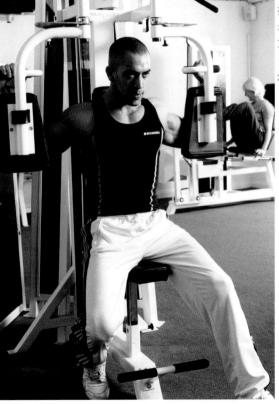

Marwood Jenkins/Alamy

Private fitness clubs generally provide high-quality facilities

Personal trainers may help individuals with low levels of fitness or self-motivation. However, such high-quality provision is too expensive for the majority, who rely instead on cheaper alternatives within the public and voluntary sectors. Sometimes individuals are deterred from private-sector participation because it is viewed as elitist and exclusively for the rich.

The key aims of private-sector provision are to:

- make a profit
- increase membership numbers
- provide an exclusive, high-quality service for members

Voluntary sector

Voluntary-sector organisations are owned and managed by members on a voluntary basis and trade on a break-even basis. For example, many local tennis clubs and rugby clubs are run by the members for the members, with any profit made being reinvested in the club, perhaps to improve facilities. Key characteristics of voluntary-sector active-leisure provision are as follows:

- clubs run by members or committees on a voluntary basis (this decreases costs and overheads)
- sometimes owned by members on a trust or charity basis
- financed by members fees, fund-raising etc.
- run on a profit-and-loss basis — making a profit is not an overriding concern

Key aims of the voluntary sector are to:

- provide for grass-roots sports participation
- increase club membership and performance levels
- provide opportunities for people to meet others with similar interests
- seek funds from sponsors and the lottery to develop playing opportunities and facilities

Best value

In the past, local-authority services and facilities for active leisure were often poorly managed with little accountability. Local taxpayers received poor value for money. A reduction in

Top tip

Exam questions sometimes require knowledge of the key characteristics of a particular sector, but often you will be asked to compare different sectors (for example, the public and private sectors). Be prepared for both types of question.

Key terms

Best value: a key government policy requiring local authorities and other related organisations to consider the best value for money they can provide. It is the principle on which local authorities decide who should run a particular service — who can provide the highest quality service at the best possible price?

Voluntary sector: local sports clubs that are often run by members or a committee.

Tasks to tackle 11.2

Give two characteristics and two objectives of voluntary-sector provision.

central government funding for active leisure provision accompanied the need for greater accountability of local authorities in relation to such provision. Local authorities therefore had to continue to meet local needs and community demands for active leisure, but increase the standards of such provision within budget, that is, break even.

'Best value' is the principle in operation in the public sector aiming to increase accountability and provide a higher quality of service for users of public-sector provision.

The main features of 'best value' are:

- consideration of best value for money
- local authorities looking to provide the best value experiences they can offer
- finding out what people want for their communities
- set standards
- services delivered to match these standards
- measuring the success of reaching the set standards

Practice makes perfect

1 Name the main sectors responsible for the provision of active leisure in the UK. *(3 marks)*

2 Facilities for active leisure are provided by a combination of private, public and voluntary sectors. Explain the main objective of each type of sector. *(3 marks)*

3 What objectives may a local authority leisure centre have that are different from those of a private health and fitness club? *(4 marks)*

Increasing participation

What you need to know

By the end of this chapter you will understand:

- the historical, social and cultural factors contributing towards the development of the current provision of PE, including the influence of the English public schools on the emergence of rational recreation (including games) and the concept of fair play
- how the development of physical activity within state elementary schools from the early twentieth century, from the concepts of military drill to post-Second World War provision and the emphasis on movement, have helped increase participation
- the characteristics of each of the key stages of the National Curriculum for PE and the relevance of each in relation to increasing opportunity for participation
- the factors influencing provision in schools and the impact this has on pupils' experiences of sport and physical activity
- the effects of developing school–club links
- initiatives such as Physical Education, School Sport and Club Link Strategy (PESSCLS), school sport coordinators (SSCOs), sports colleges, Active Sports, Sports Leaders UK, TOPS programmes of the Youth Sport Trust, Whole Sport plans designed to encourage the development of school–club links and the potential benefits to individuals, the surrounding communities and government in general
- the role of national governing bodies, Sport England and the Youth Sport Trust in raising levels of participation

Nineteenth-century public schools

Public schools were established long before state or government-provided schools were thought of. They are therefore a good place to begin our study of physical education and how the legacy of the past influences the way PE is taught in today's National Curriculum.

Public schools have a long tradition in Britain, dating back to the original nine schools of Eton, Harrow, Rugby, Charterhouse, St Paul's, Winchester, Merchant Taylors', Westminster and Shrewsbury. These schools were highly prestigious and catered for the upper classes in Victorian society, that is, those who could afford to send their sons there and who had a high social standing (the 'elite' of society).

Public school: a private, independent, fee-paying school.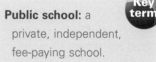

During the nineteenth century, a new social class emerged — the middle classes. They had worked hard for their new-found wealth and they wanted to emulate the lifestyles of the upper classes. They were not welcomed in the public schools established for the gentry, so they built their own proprietary colleges, such as Marlborough and Clifton.

The public schools in the nineteenth century aimed to educate the future leaders of society in their roles as politicians, lawyers and doctors, for example. Leadership skills and the behaviour befitting a gentleman were considered vital ingredients in the boys' education. Through education, the boys were taught respect for social order and were prepared to serve their country in whatever capacity was required of them.

Characteristics of public schools

Early nineteenth-century English public schools for the upper and eventually the middle classes were exclusive, elitist, fee-paying institutions for the gentry. Only a small section of society could afford to send their sons to such schools. The schools had endowed status and were controlled by trustees.

There were only a few schools, often a long way from the boys' homes and in rural locations, so most students had to board. The boys had to leave home at an early age and were institutionalised during term time for many years. The institutional lifestyle had a profound impact on the characters of the boys as they learnt their place in the hierarchical structure. The older boys became prefects in the sixth form and the younger boys — fags — were made to serve them. The bullying that arose from this situation was often harsh and frightening.

Public schools were single sex, first for the sons of the gentry and later for their daughters. Education took place in an atmosphere of strict discipline. The schools were spartan and flogging occurred frequently. The harsh treatment and basic living conditions helped to prepare the boys for adult life.

Physical activities in public schools

The boys in public schools often spent afternoons unsupervised and caused problems in local areas as they trespassed on local landowners' property, poaching and gambling. They were generally out of control. The school authorities disapproved of many of the boys' activities, because:

- they took place away from the school grounds
- they had no moral qualities
- they brought the school's reputation into disrepute

Before the 1850s, most sporting activities were actively discouraged — sport was viewed as a waste of time. In 1864, Queen Victoria appointed the Earl of Clarendon and his team of commissioners to examine all aspects of public-school life. The Clarendon report criticised many aspects and gave advice on how schools could improve. It recognised the value of team games and its legacy remains today, with games such as rugby, cricket and football in particular being popular during curricular and extra-curricular time.

Technical development and rationalisation of games

The boys began to participate in physical activities such as swimming, cross-country running, fighting and racket games. However, team games became the dominant recreational activity, largely because the schools were under pressure from the government to control the behaviour of the boys, and team games were seen as an excellent way of doing this.

Boys arriving at school from their villages brought with them numerous versions of mob games and participated in these games regularly in their spare time. Mob games were violent and disorderly; they were played by the working classes and had few rules. The masters realised the potential of these games for channelling the boys' energies and as a way of keeping them on the school grounds. The schools allowed mob games to be played only if they were given rules. Mob football underwent a number of changes as it developed towards a more rationalised activity in public schools:

- It was played more regularly, for example in games lessons.
- The boundaries were reduced — a more confined space was used.
- The numbers of players was restricted.
- The equipment and facilities became more sophisticated — actual goals were used.
- A division of labour was introduced with positional roles — people were assigned different tasks.
- Leadership roles in the form of captains were highly respected.
- A competition structure was devised, initially through the house system and later through inter-schools matches.
- Individual school rules eventually gave way to nationally recognised rules (codification).

Many public schools initially developed their own unique games, mostly as a result of the architectural features of the schools. Some of these traditions are retained, for example the Eton wall game.

A feature of the early games in public schools was that the boys organised the activities themselves. This 'self-government' gave the boys organisational skills, which they used later in life. The boys set up games committees: the hierarchical structure among the boys allowed the prefects to organise the younger boys and was seen as a form of social control.

Initially, the masters had little to do with the organisation. It was only later that 'blues' were employed as members of staff to help the school achieve victory on the playing field. 'Blues'

Task to tackle 12.1

How did English public schools influence the technical development of games?

Blues: a term used at Oxford and Cambridge universities to describe sports performers who were awarded a 'colour' for playing in the university team.

Games cult: a fanatical devotion to team games in particular and the benefits young men could get from playing them.

often returned to their old schools to coach sporting activities. By this time, the games cult and rationalisation had taken over, and headmasters used success on the sports field to impress future parents.

Fixtures were reported in the press and sports day became a public relations exercise for the 'old boys', parents and governors. Headmasters began to support the increasing use of sport by providing facilities, time and funds, as many headmasters do today.

Social control: the process whereby society seeks to ensure conformity to the dominant norms and values of that society.

Key term

Tasks to tackle 12.2

How did public schools use team games such as cricket as a form of social control?

The moral qualities assigned to team games began in the nineteenth-century public schools. The government wanted the boys' activities to be more closely supervised and orderly. At the same time, changes were taking place in society, especially the civilising and disciplining of the working classes. The middle and upper classes needed to be seen to display higher moral qualities.

Thomas Arnold, the head of Rugby School, was a major influence on reforming the public schools. His main aim was to establish social control. He encouraged team games for the moral qualities he thought the boys could gain from participating in the activities.

Arnold and his fellow public school headmasters believed that team games helped the boys to develop teamwork, loyalty, decision-making skills and leadership qualities and tested bravery and courage. The individual was not as important as the team and winning was to be sought in a sporting manner. Sportsmanship and fair play were the dominant ethos.

Athleticism and muscular Christianity

From around the middle of the nineteenth century, the cult of athleticism was evident in English public schools. Athleticism (see Table 12.1) combined **physical endeavour** (playing hard) with **moral integrity** (sportsmanship). Team games were valued for their development of character.

The movement ran parallel to the muscular Christianity movement, amateurism and Olympism. All these concepts embraced the physical and moral benefits of participating in rational sporting activities. They are viewed by some as a legacy of British sport — we continue to play down the importance of winning and instead stress that how you take part is more important. These were very much the values of the middle and upper classes in the nineteenth century and reflected a lifestyle of ease and few

Table **12.1** Athleticism

Physical endeavour	Moral integrity	Activities
Appreciation of health and fitness	Sportsmanship	Rugby
	Teamwork	Football
Toughen up an indulgent society	Honour/loyalty	Cricket
Competition in a competitive society	Leadership/response to leadership	Racquets
Combat tendency to over-study, i.e. become an all-rounder	Status held by the elite games players	

monetary worries, but they still influence the sportsmanship and fair-play ethic applied to sports participation, including school sport by many in the UK.

Muscular Christianity (see Table 12.2) was initiated by Charles Kingsley. It was an evangelical movement combining Christianity and the chivalric ideals of manliness. It included the belief that a healthy body and a healthy mind are needed in order to serve God. The muscular Christians only supported rational activities, that is, those activities that were governed by rules and codes of behaviour.

Table 12.2 A comparison of athleticism and muscular Christianity

Athleticism	Muscular Christianity
Manliness, physical robustness	Working for a team, loyalty to the cause
Pursuit of physical endeavour, effort, striving	Conforming to the rules, principle of fair play
Appreciating the value of healthy exercise and fitness	Playing honourably is more important than winning
Accepting the discipline of rule-regulated activity	Use of 'God-given' abilities
Moral integrity	Performance dedicated to God

The legacy of the nineteenth-century public schools

The National Curriculum still places a great deal of importance on team games, with the development of qualities such as sportsmanship, teamwork and leadership. Team games are still taught for their character-building qualities, and learning how to be competitive is an important part of modern life. While being competitive is important, respecting opponents and officials are key aims today, as they were in the public schools. Fair play and sportsmanship are seen as positive qualities to be developed through PE at school. Improved decision-making and cognitive skills are also seen as important values resulting from an involvement in team games.

Success in sport can raise the status of an institution and is often used as a marketing tool to promote a school. Many schools have competitive fixtures with other schools, as well as their own house systems, and some have established traditions of excellence. A number of schools have sought specialist 'sports college' status, which can further improve the sporting experiences of pupils. Sports colleges are discussed in more detail on pp. 125–126.

Development of state school education

The development of state school education is summarised in Table 12.3.

Prior to 1870, the working classes had no formal education. The Education Act was introduced in 1870. This made it compulsory for all children to attend a state school. This was not immediately popular with the working classes as it meant that the children would no longer be working and they would lose vital income.

The purpose of the state schools was to provide an education for the working classes. Many social reformers and philanthropists had worked to secure a better lifestyle for the working classes and to keep young children away from unsafe factory work. Employers needed a disciplined and educated workforce. The working classes needed to acquire basic skills — reading, writing and arithmetic. Religious education was also an important part of state education for many years as a way of instilling moral values, which the middle classes saw as being important. The working classes were going to be the factory workers, obeying commands from their employers. Discipline and obedience were therefore important values for them to learn, rather than the leadership and decision-making skills that were promoted in the public schools for the middle and upper classes.

Table 12.3 Development of state school education and physical activities

Date	Developments in state schooling	Physical activities
Pre-1870	No formal state education, some patchy church provision	—
1870	Forster Education Act, foundations of state education laid	Drill training linked to Swedish gymnastics
1899–1902	Poor performance in the Boer War put down to lack of fitness and discipline among troops	Military drill introduced via the Model Course
1902–04	War Office exercises	The Model Course delivered by NCOs
1904, 1909, 1919	Centralised government control of physical activity in state schools	Early syllabuses of physical training (PT)
1933	Last centralised syllabus of physical training	Content more varied, including gymnastics and small-sided games
1952	Influence of child-centred, self-discovery learning in primary schools	*Moving and Growing* for primary schools, followed by *Planning the Programme* in 1954
1988	Education Reform Act, National Curriculum PE introduced	Wide range of activities to be taught with attainment levels in four key stages

Characteristics of state schools

The experiences of working-class children in state schools were very different from those of the sons of the gentry in the public schools. The state schools were free of charge. They were built in local areas, as day schools, and catered for both sexes. Most age groups were taught together. Limited space with no recreational facilities imposed restrictions on the activities the state schools could offer. However, at the end of the nineteenth century it was believed that the working classes had no need of recreation.

Physical activities in state schools

Swedish gymnastics formed the basis of early state school physical activity. The Board of Education favoured the Swedish variety over the German style, which required gymnastic equipment. The Swedish system was based on therapeutic principles — a term relating to curative practices to maintain health — and scientific knowledge of the body at the time. The exercises were free standing and free flowing and taught in an instructional style.

Heavy losses suffered by Britain during the Boer War (1899–1902) were blamed on Swedish gymnastics not being rigorous enough — physically or mentally.

The Model Course

In 1902, the Model Course replaced Swedish gymnastics. The main aims of the Model Course were to improve the health and fitness of the working classes (for military service), to give training in the use of weapons, and to develop obedience and discipline in preparation for work and war.

No account was taken of the children's needs. Non-commissioned officers (NCOs) delivered military drill-style exercises taken directly from the War Office. The children were taught in a command–obey style in which the NCO adopted an authoritarian manner, making all the decisions with no input from the group. Instructions included 'Attention', 'Stand at ease', 'March', and 'About turn'. The class was taught as a group with no individual responses.

The exercises were mainly free-standing and static, and the only equipment required were sticks or staves as dummy weapons in order to teach weapon familiarity. The military drill style exercises were completed in unison.

The following are important points to note:

- Military needs became more powerful than educational theory.
- Education took a step backwards as Swedish drill, innovation and the therapeutic approach were abandoned in favour of military drill.
- Girls and boys from all age groups were instructed together.
- Children were treated as soldiers.
- The Model Course was taught by army NCOs (or teachers who had been trained by them).
- It was dull and repetitive but cheap because it catered for large numbers in a limited space.
- It lowered the status of physical activity.

> **Tasks to tackle 12.3**
>
> Contrast the ways in which the upper and middle classes were prepared for life after school with the ways in which the working classes were.

The Model Course lasted for just 2 years because it had no educational focus, it did not cater for children's needs and its intention of improving the health and fitness of the children was questionable.

Syllabuses of physical training (1904–33)

The Model Course was replaced by the 1904 syllabus of physical training. The government produced a prescriptive syllabus that could be delivered by teachers with no previous experience of teaching physical training. The syllabus stressed the physical and educative effects of sporting activities and emphasised the benefits of exercise in the open air. However, schools still had limited facilities and the working classes were still required to be obedient. The style of teaching was similar to drill but without the military content.

Changes occurred gradually over a number of years. The last PT syllabus in 1933 involved more free movement, more creativity and some group work. Children were increasingly encouraged to use their imagination and there was a greater focus on the development of skills. There was growing interaction between teachers and pupils, and the influence of specialist teachers trained in the techniques of Rudolf Laban was felt. Laban was a dancer, a choreographer and a dance/movement theoretician. His work in the late 1930s and after the Second World War led to more progressive teaching methods and child-centred teaching through activities such as dance.

> **Child-centred:** basing a programme of study around a child's physical, cognitive, social and emotional needs.

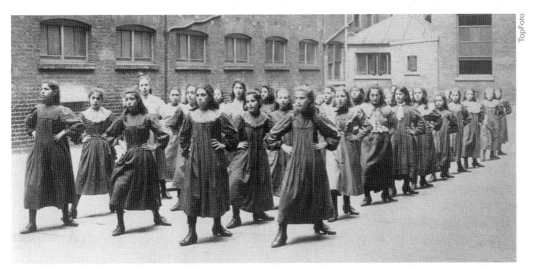

Girls exercising at school during the early 1900s

Early developments in physical training syllabuses

The key objectives of the early syllabuses (1904–09) were the therapeutic effects of exercise, with emphasis on respiration, circulation and posture. Obedience and discipline were still important but enjoyment started to appear as an aim in lessons. Alertness, decision-making and control of mind over body began to feature.

Dr George Newman was a key influence on the development of PT syllabuses. He was appointed as Chief Medical Officer within the Board of Education. As a doctor, he was interested in the health-giving effects of exercise.

The 1904 syllabus comprised 109 'tables' of exercises for teachers to follow. The introduction of the 1909 syllabus saw this reduced to 71 tables. Teaching methods still included commands delivered to children in ranks, with marching and free-standing exercises but also allowed a kinder approach by teachers and some freedom of choice. The 1909 syllabus was more Swedish in character, with recreational aspects to relieve the tedium and monotony of former drill-style lessons. Dancing steps and simple games were introduced.

The 1919 syllabus

Set against the huge losses of life from the First World War and as a result of the post-war flu epidemic, the 1919 syllabus was progressive in terms of its broader content and more child-centred approach.

Dr George Newman was still influential and eager to refute accusations that PT was to blame for the lack of fitness among the working classes. He also stressed the benefits of recreational activities for the rehabilitation of injured soldiers.

The main objectives of the 1919 PT syllabus were enjoyment and play for the under-7s and therapeutic work for the over-7s. This was the first time age differentiation had appeared in PT lessons.

The exercises were similar to those of the 1909 syllabus (free-standing) with a special section of games for the under-7s. It was recommended that at least half the lesson should be spent on 'general activity exercises' such as active free movement, to include small games and dancing.

Teachers were given more freedom to deliver lessons in a less formal way and to give children a varied physical experience.

The 1933 syllabus

The industrial depression of the 1930s left many of the working class unemployed and living in poverty (no state benefits were available at this time).

A new syllabus of physical training introduced in 1933 was seen as a watershed between the syllabuses of the past and the physical education of the future. It was more varied in its aims, content and teaching methodology than earlier syllabuses, and included one section for the under-11s and one for the over-11s. This development followed the Hadow Report of 1926, which identified the continuing need to differentiate between ages for physical training.

This was the last syllabus to be published under the direction of Dr George Newman. It is important to note that the 1933 PT syllabus was a detailed, high-quality and highly respected syllabus.

The syllabus was still set out as a series of tables, which teachers used to plan their lessons. The emphasis was still on physical fitness, therapeutic results, good posture and physique. The syllabus included athletics, gymnastics and games skills as well as group work. Development of both mind and body (that is, holistic development) was a key aim.

The style of teaching was still direct for most of the lesson but some decentralised work was included, in which the teacher acted as a guide and the children worked at their own pace to solve problems. Group work was a main feature. Many schools now had specialist facilities such as newly built gymnasiums. Special clothing was worn during lessons.

Tasks to tackle 12.4

What were the main differences between the early syllabuses of physical training (1904–09) and the final syllabus in 1933 in terms of content and delivery?

Development of PE in the 1950s

The influence of the Second World War

The development of state PE in the 1950s coincided with an extensive post-war rebuilding programme — many schools were destroyed during the Second World War. This led to an expansion in the facilities available to deliver a more varied physical education programme than existed at the start of the century.

The apparatus brought into schools after the war was a direct result of the commando training that had taken place during the war. Troops needed to engage in a more mobile style of fighting and to be able to solve problems. The educational value of this type of activity was recognised and different styles of teaching emerged in order to develop children in a more positive way while recognising their physical, mental, social and emotional needs.

Rudolf Laban influenced the development of state PE in the 1950s with his work on movement to music, educational dance and creativity. His work was influential in *Moving and Growing* (1952) and *Planning the Programme* (1954).

Moving and Growing (1952) and *Planning the Programme* (1954)

The (Butler) Education Act 1944 aimed to ensure equality of educational opportunity. The school leaving age was raised to 15 years and local authorities were required to provide playing fields for all schools.

PE in the 1950s aimed to develop physical, social and cognitive skills, to provide a variety of experiences in an enjoyable atmosphere, with increased involvement for everyone at their own level of ability. It included agility exercises, gymnastics, dance and games skills, swimming and movement to music.

The teaching style was child-centred, enjoyment-orientated and progressive. Teachers guided rather than directed. Individual interpretation of tasks was encouraged, leading to a problem-solving, creative, exploratory, discovery style of learning. Apparatus such as ropes, bars, boxes and mats was used in lessons.

Moving and Growing was published by the Education Department as a guide for primary schools. Primary school teachers were not trained specifically in physical education so needed guidance to plan and deliver it. The term 'physical education' had now evolved, giving it a very different emphasis from the earlier 'physical training'. Immediately, it suggested that there was now a belief that the mind needed to be involved as well as the body. This was combined with the movement approach and saw the following developments in PE teaching:

- exploratory work
- problem solving
- creativity
- skill-based work

These developments reflected changes in educational thinking. There was now a more child-centred approach, with teachers being able to show initiative and autonomy. The teaching style changed from a command–obey style to a more heuristic style (in which pupils discovered or

Tasks to tackle 12.5

Describe the content and teaching style of the *Moving and Growing* programme.

reached an understanding through exploratory work or trial and error). The problems had open-ended possibilities rather than predetermined goals set by adults; therefore a sense of success was more likely to occur. A guidance style of teaching, where the children were given a stimulus to which they responded through movement within their own capabilities, was also used, particularly in dance and educational gymnastics.

The start of a 'recreational focus'

In the last decades of the twentieth century, radical changes were made to physical activities in state schools. The Butler Education Act 1944 required local authorities to provide recreational sporting facilities in schools. This was a very different philosophy from the one held at the beginning of the twentieth century, which believed that the working classes had no need for recreation. The secondary school teacher was now fully trained and therefore was no longer dependent on following a syllabus drawn up centrally. Physical education teachers were to experience about 40 years of a decentralised system where they had autonomy and were able to choose their own physical education programmes.

National Curriculum PE

By the end of the 1980s the government wanted:
- more control of education
- more teacher accountability
- national standards for physical education
- a wider range of activities to be taught

> **Key term**
>
> **Centralised:** to draw under central control — the government directs policy across a country to seek uniformity.

The 1988 Education Reform Act led to the introduction of National Curriculum physical education, which applies to all state schools. This represented a return to a centralised approach towards education. All state schools now follow set guidelines for set subjects and are inspected by Ofsted.

The status of PE was reinforced by making it compulsory for all 5–16-year-olds. The aims of National Curriculum PE are given on pp. 100–101. Through physical education, children should be able to:
- achieve physical competence, that is, improve physical skills
- improve self-confidence and knowledge of strengths and weaknesses
- perform in a range of activities including those that encourage active leisure time
- improve health and fitness
- become a 'critical performer', that is, children should be encouraged to observe and analyse physical activities in a knowledgeable way
- learn how to plan, perform and evaluate
- improve cognitive skills and decision-making
- improve social skills and leadership qualities

Key functions of the National Curriculum

Therapeutic functions

One of the main aims of the PE National Curriculum is to raise awareness in children of the need for a healthy lifestyle. Modern life tends to encourage children to be more sedentary; active play has been reduced in favour of the television and computer games. Increased safety concerns have led to fewer children walking to school than in earlier generations, and the fast-food culture is leading to an increasing problem of obesity, which affects individuals and society alike.

Creativity

Since the middle of the twentieth century, children have been required by educationists to be more creative and imaginative in their PE lessons. The National Curriculum has given creativity even more importance through formal assessment.

Recreational breadth

The range of physical activities taught in schools has gradually increased over the last 50 years. In trying to combat the problem of teachers offering only a few activities, the National Curriculum has made this a formal requirement. Schools have developed better facilities, greater use has been made of community facilities, and since the

TopFoto

Schools now offer a range of physical activities, including team sports

1970s there has been a policy of educating people to use their leisure time effectively. The idea is that the more activities you experience, the more likely you are to find one that you enjoy and will carry on into later life. This brings benefits to individuals and to society.

Critical performer

The National Curriculum aims to provide people with knowledge of roles in sport other than performer. Roles such as official, coach, spectator and leader encourage children to appreciate physical activities in different ways, and possibly to take on some of these roles at various stages of their lives.

Areas of activity

The current aims of PE are to offer a broad range of physical activities. Concentrating on one activity would not provide a balanced physical development. The National Curriculum classifications are:

- games
- athletic activities
- swimming
- gymnastics
- dance
- outdoor and adventurous activities (OAA)

Schools cannot offer every sport available but there should be a balance of activities — team and individual, competitive and non-competitive — selected from the six categories listed.

Structure of the National Curriculum

There are four key stages with eight levels of attainment. Key Stages 1 and 2 are primary school levels; Key Stages 3 and 4 are for secondary schools.

Key Stage 1 is for 5–7-year-olds. It offers a limited range of activities and no choice. Pupils are required to study three areas: gymnastics, games and dance. The aim is to develop simple skills and eventually sequences of movement, independently and then with a partner. Pupils are taught about changes that occur to their bodies when they exercise and to recognise the short-term effects of exercise on the body.

Key Stage 2, for 7–11-year-olds, allows development of individual skills in isolation and of simple skills. Six areas should be studied: games, gymnastics and dance are compulsory; the other areas include athletic activities, outdoor and adventurous activities, and swimming and water safety. Pupils should improve their motor skills and coordination, develop more complex patterns of movement, sustain energetic activity and understand the effects of exercise.

Primary school teachers are not usually specialists in physical education, although specialist help is often sought for swimming classes. In recent years, national governing bodies such as the Lawn Tennis Association and the Rugby Football Union have begun to tap into primary schools using coaches funded by lottery money to initiate interest within schools. In order to access extra lottery funding, the governing bodies have to highlight in their policies and plans how they intend to increase participation at the grass-roots level of sport. These initiatives are often optional, but they do increase the range of activities offered in schools and raise awareness of sport among young children.

At this stage, children are learning the fundamental motor skills they will require in more specific sporting situations and therefore it is important that they receive the best teaching possible. The TOPs programme, run by the Youth Sport Trust, and specialist sports colleges and school sport coordinators contribute to the experiences offered at primary schools.

Key Stage 3 is taught to children aged 11–14 years. A wider range of activities is on offer at secondary school. Pupils at this stage should be refining their motor skills, undertaking more complex movements, and beginning to learn rules and tactics and how to recover after activity.

Teachers delivering lessons at Key Stage 3 should aim to:

- develop physical skills such as running, jumping and landing
- develop social skills and communication skills
- improve creativity and imagination
- develop problem-solving skills
- create a safe working environment
- meet National Curriculum objectives
- allow individuals to reach their potential in a fun learning environment

Key Stage 4, for 14–16-year-olds, requires a choice of activities and the opportunity to start specialising. Pupils should be prepared to plan, undertake and evaluate a safe, health-promoting exercise programme and show understanding of the principles involved. Experiencing a variety of roles other than performing is important at this stage. The development of more complex and advanced skills in competitive situations becomes important.

Secondary school NC PE programmes of study from September 2008

QCA guidelines (see www.qca.org.uk/curriculum) for schools and PE teachers recommend that at Key Stage 3 at least four areas of activity from the list outlined below should be experienced, with more specialisation in two activities from the list at Key Stage 4.

The range and content for PE teachers to select from is:

- outwitting opponents, as in games activities
- accurate replication of actions, phrases and sequences, as in gymnastics activities
- exploring and communicating ideas, concepts and emotions, as in dance activities
- performing at maximum levels in relation to speed, height, distance, strength or accuracy, as in athletics activities
- identifying and solving problems to overcome challenges of an adventurous nature, as in life saving and personal survival in swimming and outdoor activities
- exercising safely and effectively to improve health and well-being, as in fitness and health activities

Factors influencing PE and sport provision in schools

A pupil's experience of PE and sport at school can be positive or negative, depending on various factors in individual schools.

Timetable restrictions

Schools sometimes reduce the amount of time allocated to PE/sport due to the demands of other, 'more academic' subjects. PE may be marginalised, particularly at Key Stage 4 when the demands of GCSE examinations are high.

Lack of funding or resources

Budgets may restrict the quality and breadth of a pupil's PE experience. Many schools find the funding of swimming and OAA particularly difficult. Transport for fixtures might also be deemed too expensive and negatively affect inter-school sporting opportunities.

Quality of staffing

PE teachers and external coaches vary in terms of qualifications and degree of commitment to PE/school sport, and this may affect the quality of a pupil's early physical activity experience.

Quality of facilities

The availability of specialist facilities for offering a range of PE and sport varies throughout the country.

School–club links

Links between schools and clubs can positively influence PE and school sport by improving a pupil's access to high-quality coaching and facilities.

Assessment

Each key stage has an end-of-key-stage description. Teachers record pupils' planning, performance and evaluation. Teachers have to indicate whether the pupil is working beyond, at the level of, or towards the end-of-key-stage description. While recognising the need for assessment, some teachers are concerned that the amount of assessment can be overdone (see Table 12.4). Attainment targets are set for the four key stages where children are assessed on their knowledge, skills and understanding in the areas of activity experienced. The purpose of attainment targets is to set general expectations of what children should be able to accomplish by the end of each stage.

Table 12.4 Advantages and disadvantages of National Curriculum PE assessment

Advantages of assessment	Disadvantages of assessment
Clear objectives and goals to reach	Too much time spent on testing
Gives incentives/rewards and motivation to improve	Tests are mainly subjective
Improves quality of teaching	Not every child can achieve the highest levels
Gives recognition to good teachers	Can demotivate teachers and children due to unfair comparisons
	Too much pressure takes away the fun element

School sport

As well as the core curriculum lessons, children are offered many other sporting experiences at school. Extra-curricular activities are optional activities offered in schools during lunchtime and after school. They offer recreational experiences as well as competitive fixtures. This is also called **school sport**, which should be differentiated from physical education. Physical education refers to the compulsory core lessons. There is an overlap between school sport and physical education but their central focus is different. Physical education provides the building blocks for the extra-curricular programmes that will enhance and extend a child's interest and aptitude. One problem is that extra-curricular activities rely on the goodwill of teachers and this is not always forthcoming.

In the 1980s, there was a decline in the extra-curricular opportunities offered to children in the state-school sector. Many factors affected the downturn in competitive school sports:

- teacher strikes based on contractual hours reduced teachers' goodwill
- financial pressures of running fixtures
- the competing leisure and employment options of teenagers
- the anti-competitive lobby was against inter-school sport

In the UK, physical education and school sport have traditionally been kept separate, as they are believed to serve different aims. However, there is now a growing belief that these two strands should be brought closer together and initiatives are taking place to try to achieve this. Examples include the Physical Education, School Sport and Club Links (PESSCL) strategy and sports college status being given to some schools.

Current government policies

PE, School Sport and Club Links (PESSCL) strategy

PESSCL has a number of 'sub-programmes' that you need to be familiar with, for example sports colleges, school sport partnerships, Step into Sport and Club Links.

The Sport England website reports government investment to deliver the PESSCL strategy of £978 million between 2003 and 2008:

www.sportengland.org/index/get_resources/schoolsport/pesscl.htm

PESSCL is a national strategy aimed at increasing the uptake of sporting opportunities by 5–16-year-olds so that 85% of them experience a minimum of 2 hours of high-quality PE and school sport each week. It is delivered through nine interlinked strands:

- sports colleges
- school sport partnerships
- professional development
- Step into Sport
- Club Links
- Gifted and Talented
- sporting playgrounds
- swimming
- the QCA's PE and School Sport Investigation

Sports colleges

Sports colleges are part of the specialist schools programme, which is run by the Department for Children, Schools and Families (formerly the Department for Education and Skills, DfES).

Sports colleges help to deliver the government's plans for PE and sport. They provide high-quality opportunities for young people in their neighbourhood.

Sport is one of ten specialisms within the specialist schools programme. The programme helps schools to establish a distinctive identity through their chosen specialism. Sports colleges aim to raise standards of achievement in PE and sport for all their students. They are regional focal points for:

- promoting excellence in PE and sport in the community
- extending links between families of schools, sports bodies and communities, sharing resources and developing and sharing good practice
- helping young people to progress to careers in sport and PE

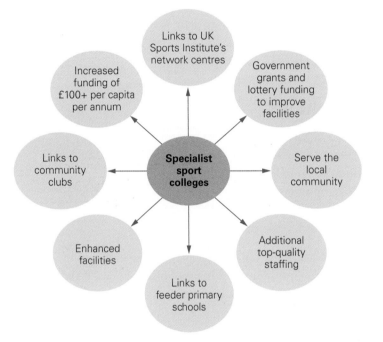

Key terms

Sports colleges: part of the government's specialist schools programme; sports colleges are secondary schools that have achieved specialist status for sport.

School sport partnerships: secondary schools linked to a 'cluster' of primary schools, for example to provide sports competitions.

Top tip

E-mail ystinfo@lboro.ac.uk to find out what is happening in your area.

Figure 12.1 Features of specialist sports colleges

School sport partnerships

School sport partnerships are groups of schools that receive funding from the government to come together to enhance sporting opportunities. There are 450 partnerships across schools in England. Each partnership is individual but a 'partnership model' has been devised to develop new partnerships and expand existing ones (Figure 12.2).

The aims of a school sport partnership team are to:

- enhance opportunities for young people to experience different sports
- access high-quality coaching
- engage in competition

Typically, partnerships:

- are clustered around a specialist sports college and managed by a full-time **partnership development manager**, whose role is to develop links with the LEA, other sports organisations and the wider community
- include around eight secondary school partners, each of which appoints a **school sport coordinator** (SSCo). SSCos are PE teachers who are released from the timetable for 2 days each week to work with their cluster of primary schools, developing after-school activities and links with the local community and sports clubs.

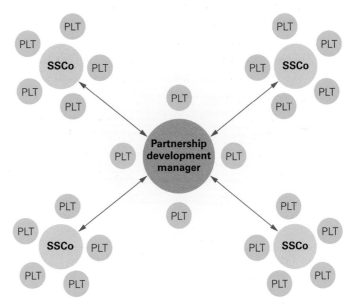

Figure 12.2 School sport partnerships (SSCo, school sport coordinator; PLT, primary link teacher)

- include around 45 primary or special school partners (clustered in families of five around the sports college and secondary schools), each of which appoints a **primary link teacher** who is released from timetable for 12 days each year to help develop PE and school sport within the primary school

The overall aim of the partnerships is to help schools to enable their pupils to spend at least 2 hours each week on high-quality PE and school sport. Six objectives have been set to help achieve this aim:

- strategic planning — develop and implement a PE/sport strategy
- primary liaison — develop links, particularly between Key Stages 2 and 3
- out-of-school hours — provide enhanced opportunities for all pupils
- school to community — increase participation in community sport
- coaching and leadership — provide opportunities in leadership, coaching and officiating for senior pupils, teachers and other adults
- raising standards of pupil achievement

The quality and amount of school sport is rising each year. In September 2004, the prime minister, Tony Blair, announced that **competition managers** would be added to the network of school sport partnerships. As a result of investment from the PESSCL strategy, the first 20 competition managers took up post in September 2005. Their role is to plan, manage and implement a programme of inter-school competition across their school sport partnership and others.

The Youth Sport Trust, Sport England and the National Council for School Sport have developed a framework to complement the principles of athlete development in the long term. It aims to provide consistency in competition structure for the following:

- Key Stage 3–4 (ages 12–16), inter-school leagues and cup competitions
- Key Stage 3 (ages 11–12), multi-sport competition, central venue leagues
- Key Stage 2 (ages 9–11), multi-sport competition, central venue leagues
- Key Stage 2 (ages 7–9), multi-skill festivals each term
- Key Stage 1 (ages 4–7), annual multi-skill festivals (off-site)

Each national governing body (NGB) is working closely with its National Schools Association to develop a new, integrated structure of competitions, from inter-school (local) to inter-district (county level) and above, using the new families of schools as geographic units for competition.

Step into Sport

Step into Sport and Club Links are the key strands of PESSCL that aim to provide the links from high-quality school sport to high-quality community sport, and to ensure that all young people have the best possible experience either as a participant or as a volunteer.

> **Key term**
>
> **Step into Sport:** a Youth Sport Trust scheme to increase the number of sports leaders in the 14–19 age range.

Step into Sport is part of the National School Sport Strategy, which was produced jointly by the Department for Culture, Media and Sport and the DfES. It is managed by Sport England and the Youth Sport Trust with Sports Leaders UK and provides a high-quality sports leadership training service. School sport partnerships work with county sport partnerships and national governing bodies of sport to target 14–19-year-olds by providing opportunities for young people to get involved in leadership and volunteering in sport.

The community volunteering aspect of Step into Sport enables 16–19-year-olds to take part in a range of activities staged by sports clubs and other organisations. Young people can play a variety of roles, including managing events and facilities, media duties and running a club, as well as assistant coach or referee roles. The aim is to support young volunteers in developing key life skills and in gaining new skills, knowledge, self-confidence and qualifications.

Club Links

A school–club link is an agreement between a school or a school sport partnership and a community-based sports club to work together to meet the needs of all young people who might want to get involved in their sport/club. It helps young people to realise their ambitions in sport and dance by providing pathways for them to follow. A school–club link can provide new and varied opportunities for people and put in place quality controls to ensure that standards remain high.

The main aim of the Club Links programme is to increase the number of children participating in sports clubs. A target was set to increase the percentage of 5–16-year-olds who were members of sports clubs from 14% in 2002 to 25% by 2008. The PESSCL survey for 2004–05 showed that an average of 22% of pupils in school sport partnerships participated in at least one sports club with links to the school, surpassing the 2006 target of 20%.

Twenty-two NGBs receive funding to work with and support their accredited clubs and help them to make sustainable and effective links with schools by working in partnership with county and school sport partnerships.

Progress has already been made with this scheme, including 800 multi-skill clubs being set up for primary school children in the 7–11 age range. Delivered through the network of school sport partnerships, these clubs provide additional opportunities for children to develop fundamental motor and movement skills, and act as a stepping stone into club sport.

> **Top tip**
>
> For more information on multi-skill clubs see www.youthsporttrust.org/linkAttachments/scuk-multi-skils-faqs.pdf

Dance Links

Dance Links is a dance-specific project within Club Links. Its aim is to help improve links between school sport partnerships and dance providers to increase the number of young people participating in dance. Dance Links is also working to enhance the choice and quality of children's dance experience to increase the likelihood of maintaining their lifelong participation in this area.

> **Tasks to tackle 12.6**
>
> How can schools and community sports clubs work together to increase the levels of participation in sport and recreation?

NGBs and whole sport plans

In 2003, Sport England identified 30 priority sports, based on their ability to contribute to Sport England's vision of an active and successful sporting nation. Sport England is working with the NGBs of these sports to develop and implement their whole sport plans (WSPs).

Whole sport plans identify how a sport will contribute to Sport England's 'start', 'stay' and 'succeed' objectives from grass roots through to elite level. The plans identify what help and resources NGBs need to deliver their whole sport plans. They enable Sport England to direct funding and resources to NGBs and offer the opportunity to measure how well the NGBs are performing.

Seven key performance indicators (KPIs) have been agreed that reflect proposals and feedback from Sport England, UK Sport, NGBs and other relevant partners. These link to Sport England's 'start', 'stay' and 'succeed' objectives (p. 130):

- participation — an increase in participation through NGB-driven activity
- clubs — more accredited clubs within the sport
- membership — more active members of clubs within the sport
- coaches — more qualified coaches and instructors delivering instruction in the sport
- volunteers — more active volunteers supporting the sport

- international athletes — improved performance by teams and/or individuals in significant international championships and world rankings
- English athletes representing GB — a higher percentage of English athletes in GB teams in sports competing as GB

Increasing participation

NGBs are required to open their sport to all sections of society, including those at grass-roots participation levels. Ways of achieving increased participation and sports equity include:

- developing policies linking to specific target groups, for example disabled and ethnic minorities
- training more sport-specific coaches to encourage participation
- developing mini-games and modified versions of their sports to encourage participation at all levels of ability, for example high 5 netball and short tennis
- making facilities more accessible, affordable and attractive, targeting funds at grass-roots levels and inner-city schemes
- improving awareness of the sport through publicity, advertising and use of positive role models

Sport England

Sport England has a Royal Charter, which means that although it is free from political control, it is still accountable for its actions. It is a government-funded agency with responsibility for 'creating an active nation through sport'. Sport England views its primary role as sustaining and increasing participation in community sport.

SPORT ENGLAND

The key objectives of Sport England are for people to:

- **start** — increase participation in sport by 1% annually, to improve the nation's health (particularly in various target groups such as women and ethnic minorities)
- **stay** — retain people in sport, and increase club membership and numbers receiving coaching
- **succeed** — become the 'best' nation in the world by 2020 in terms of participation

Sport England is therefore trying to sustain and increase participation in community sport by promoting, investing in and advising on high-quality sports pathways that release potential through community sports activities, sports clubs, coaches and officiating and sports facilities.

Sport England makes an important contribution to the success of raising participation in school sport. A target was set to ensure that by 2008 at least 85% of school-aged children spend a minimum of 2 hours each week on high-quality PE and school sport. Sport England has a particular role to play in supporting the 2-hour 'community element' of the 2010 target minimum of 4 hours of sport offered to children. The target is measured annually through the National School Sport Survey. Sport England's contribution

Top tip

Sport England does not build sports facilities but it does improve them by investing lottery funds.

focuses on the school–club links, Step into Sport and competition managers strands within the National School Sport Strategy. Data published in October 2006 showed that good progress is being made.

Sport England's target of increasing participation in sport for 2 million people by 2012 is divided between nine regional sports boards in England. Regional sports boards work with the county sports partnerships and community sports networks in their regions.

Their role is to deliver government aims for sport in their regions and allocate resources given to them with maximum effectiveness.

The Youth Sport Trust and UK Sport

All these organisations are aiming to ensure smooth pathways to releasing the sporting potential (including volunteering, coaching, effective leadership and officiating) of as many people as possible.

YOUTH SPORT TRUST

- The Youth Sport Trust is primarily responsible for sustaining and increasing the quality and quantity of school sport (including curriculum PE).
- Sport England is primarily responsible for sustaining and increasing participation in formal and informal community sport.
- UK Sport is primarily responsible for the development and performance of world-class elite athletes (this will be explored more in Unit 3 at A2).

Historically, the transition from school sport to elite-level sport has not always been as smooth as the organisations would have wanted. This is shown by the massive decline in sport participation that occurs at 16, that is, the 'post-school gap' (see pp. 135–136), and the difficulties some elite athletes from more deprived backgrounds face in getting to the podium. In order to make the transition from school sport to community sport smoother, Sport England needs to run alongside the Youth Sport Trust ahead of the handover at 16. Sport England's role in this area is to ensure through its work with sports nationally, regionally and locally that the sporting environment is attractive and supportive of young people. This will help to ensure that they stay in sport once they leave compulsory schooling. Attempts to ensure this are through:

- club development — making sure clubs are strong enough to reach out to schools and young people
- community sports provision — including non-sports youth clubs such as the Scouts
- helping NGBs develop effective competition frameworks for children and young people
- the development of NGB volunteering strategies for young people

Sport England therefore has a crucial role to play in the Club Links, competition managers and Step into Sport strands of the National School Sport Strategy. It also has an important role to play in linking with UK Sport's World Class Performance Programme. Sport England is responsible for funding elite sport for non-Olympic sports such as squash and netball. It also funds the Commonwealth Games Council of England. Sport England sees such links to elite sport as 'a modest element' of its role.

Tasks to tackle 12.7

Name three policies that Sport England has developed to encourage increased participation in sport.

Get Active/Active Sports programme

Active Sports is a scheme coordinated by Sport England based on the following policies:

- Active Schools forms the foundation.
- Active Communities looks at breaking down the barriers to participation and considers sports equity issues.
- Active Sports — Sport England has targeted nine sports, including girls' football and rugby league, through which it hopes to encourage more young people to take part in, improve through and benefit from extra-curricular involvement. It links participation to excellence, for example via the Millennium Youth Games, and encourages those interested in taking part in a sport to join a club.

Activemark, Sportsmark and Sports Partnership Mark

In 2004, Sport England was involved in discussions with government departments on proposals to develop and reintroduce from 2006 Activemark, Sportsmark and the new Sports Partnership Mark. The key changes were as follows:

- Delivery of kitemark rewards by the national PESSCL strategy. This means that only schools within a school sport partnership are eligible.
- The kitemarks are awarded annually through the National School Sport Survey, which all partnership schools take part in.

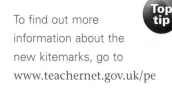

To find out more information about the new kitemarks, go to www.teachernet.gov.uk/pe

Sports Leaders UK

Sports Leaders UK provides the opportunity and motivation for people to make a meaningful contribution to their local community through nationally recognised Sports Leader Awards.

Following the award of various government grants to encourage participation in volunteering, Sports Leaders UK has developed its partnerships with organisations working with young people in the 14–19 age range. It is involved in the Step into Sport initiative, working with the Youth Sport Trust and Sport England to train a new generation of volunteer coaches, mainly in this 14–19 age range.

Sports Leaders UK is responsible for:

- the Junior Sports Leadership Award for 14–16 year olds, taught mainly within the National Curriculum for PE at Key Stage 4. The award develops young people's skills in organising activities, planning, communicating and motivating.

- the Community Sports Leadership Award, designed for the 16+ age group and delivered in a range of institutions such as schools, colleges, youth clubs and sports centres
- the Higher Sports Leadership Award, which builds on the skills gained through the Community Sports Leadership Award to equip people to lead specific community groups such as the elderly, people with disabilities and children of primary school age
- the Basic Expedition Leadership Award, designed for people interested in the outdoors, which develops the ability to organise safe expeditions and overnight camps.

The core values of these awards include:
- developing leadership — teaching people how to organise activities, and to lead, motivate and communicate with groups
- developing skills for life
- providing a stepping stone to employment as they offer a recognised qualification
- encouraging volunteering in communities
- reducing youth crime
- supporting more active, healthier communities, by providing sports leaders to organise a range of physical activity sessions

The Youth Sport Trust

The Youth Sport Trust is the key organisation with responsibility for developing school sport. It works with a range of partners such as Sport England and Sports Leaders UK.

The Youth Sport Trust believes strongly in the power of sport to improve the lives of young people. It believes that all youngsters should receive an introduction to PE and sport that links to their developmental needs. They should be able to experience and enjoy PE and sport as a result of high-quality teaching, coaching, equipment and resources.

The Youth Sport Trust is involved in a number of initiatives to help achieve these aims.

TOP programmes

These are a series of linked, progressive schemes for people aged from 18 months to 18 years. Over 20 000 schools are involved in TOP programmes such as:
- TOP Tots — helping young children aged from 18 months to 3 years experience physical activities and games
- TOP Start — encouraging 3–5-year-olds to learn through physical activity
- TOP Play — supporting 4–9-year-olds as they acquire and develop core skills
- TOP Sport — providing 7–11-year-olds with opportunities to develop skills in a range of sports
- TOP Skill — allowing 11–14-year-olds to extend their sports skills and knowledge
- TOP Link — encouraging links between schools and encouraging 14–16-year-olds to organise and manage sport and dance festivals in local primary schools and special schools — this is part of the Step into Sport programme and is also connected to the Junior Sports Leadership and Community Sports Leadership awards

- TOP Sportsability in creating opportunities for young disabled people to enjoy, participate and perform in sport

PESSCL

The Youth Sport Trust plays a central role in supporting the government's PESSCL strategy and its key aim of increasing sports activity among 5–16-year-olds. As part of the strategy, the Youth Sport Trust works with a range of partners, including government agencies, to support the development of specialist sports colleges (for example, by assisting schools in every aspect of the application process and working with schools to realise their potential on achieving sports college status) and school sport partnerships.

> ## Task to tackle 12.8
>
> TOP Sport is an example of a primary school PE initiative designed to improve the quality of a pupil's experience. Describe the key features of TOP Sport.

Step into Sport pathway

The Youth Sport Trust also plays an important role in the Step into Sport programme.

- Step 1: young people engage in a programme of sports education at school.
- Step 2: young people move on to undertake the nationally recognised Level 1 Sports Leader Award.
- Step 3: young people gain practical experience in volunteering through planning and running a TOP Link sports festival for primary-school-aged children.
- Step 4: young people undertake accredited community sports leadership training and sport-specific leadership training.
- Step 5: young people, supported by a teacher mentor, engage in a programme of volunteering in their local community. County sport partnerships help to ensure that volunteering opportunities are available, appropriate and of high quality.

UK Ambassadors

Eight hundred young ambassadors are being appointed to spread the Olympic message and to act as role models for other young people.

Each school sport partnership nominates two young people. One is a 'gifted and talented' young athlete, the other a young sports leader or volunteer. Selection takes place in Year 11, although the majority of their role is undertaken in Year 12.

Talent Matters project

The Talent Matters website gives gifted young sports people access to comprehensive information, advice and support. It is a key part of the Youth Sport Trust's Gifted and Talented programme, which is part of the government's overall PESSCL strategy.

For more information on the Talent Matters project, go to: www.talentmatters.org

School Sport Champion

Kelly Holmes was appointed School Sport Champion to encourage and promote achievement in competitive school sport, which is a key aim of the Youth Sport Trust's work.

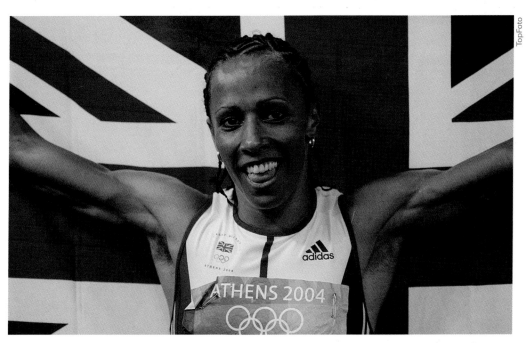

Double Olympic gold winner Kelly Holmes, Athens 2004

The post-school gap

The fall in sports participation with age mentioned earlier in this chapter is worrying because individuals reduce their chances of maintaining health and agility and of being able to live independently into their old age. Research shows that people who are exposed to a wide range of sporting activities in their youth are more likely to continue to participate throughout their lives.

There is a huge drop in participation when young people leave school — the 'post-school gap'. This drop is higher in the UK than in some other European countries and has concerned the government and sporting institutions for many decades.

Lifelong learning is a government policy that aims to enable people to take part in physical activities that will enrich their lives, and the community, for a long time. Traditionally, school PE programmes have involved team games, but research suggests that people give up these activities as they get older. In the last decades of the twentieth century, schools began to branch out and offer other activities, sometimes using community facilities to promote the opportunities available to young people in their wider community. Activities such as golf, bowls, badminton and swimming are sporting activities that people can continue with for the rest of their lives.

Table 12.5 The post-school gap

Reasons for the post-school gap	Solutions to the post-school gap
Physical education is no longer compulsory	Improve links between schools and clubs so that continued participation is more likely
Young adults have competing leisure interests	Develop knowledge about the need for a healthy lifestyle
Facilities are no longer as accessible or free to use	Offer concessionary rates to young people with a limited disposable income
Traditionally poor links between schools and clubs	Youth sections at clubs linked to schools (e.g. share facilities, coaches)

If the youth section drops out of society, the social consequences are costly. Sport is seen as one way of including young people in positive activities, channelling their energies, and making them less likely to resort to drugs and alcohol. Sport can help them to acquire new skills and integrate into wider society.

> **Tasks to tackle 12.9**
>
> Why can golf be considered a lifelong sport?

Schools have been challenging the idea of teaching only the traditional activities and, with the help of national governing bodies, they are trying to introduce new sports into their curriculum. Adaptations in equipment and the development of mini-games have meant that more activities are suitable for teaching in schools.

Reasons for government emphasis on PE and school sport

The government believes in the power of PE and sport to improve and enrich people's quality of life, to raise their self-esteem and confidence levels, as well as to provide enjoyment to individuals in society.

PE/sport is seen as having an important role to play in building stronger, safer communities, strengthening the economy and developing the skills of local people. It also meets the needs of improving the health and fitness of individuals and society in general. Coming into power in 2007, Prime Minister Gordon Brown announced a £100 million campaign to give every child the chance of 5 hours of sport every week. He called for a united effort in the run-up to the 2012 Olympics to make sport a part of every child's day, so that we can build a 'greater and fitter' sporting nation. His new plans include greater emphasis on competition within and between schools, a network of competition managers and a new National School Sports Week.

The £100 million will fund:

- provision of up to 5 hours of sport per week for all pupils and 3 hours for young people aged 16–19
- a new National School Sports Week, championed by Dame Kelly Holmes, when all schools will be encouraged to run sports days and inter-school tournaments — this is designed to build on the success of the UK School Games and motivate young people to take part in competitive sport
- a network of 225 competition managers across the country to work with primary and secondary schools to increase the amount of competitive sport they offer
- more coaches in schools and the community to deliver expert advice to young people

Practice makes perfect

1 The Model Course (1902–04) was introduced into state elementary schools as a result of poor performance in the Boer War. What were the objectives of the Model Course?

(2 marks)

2 How did the change in content and teaching style of the programme *Moving and Growing* reflect the changing attitude towards children in the mid-twentieth century? *(3 marks)*

3 Give two ways in which National Curriculum PE encourages pupils to develop an appreciation of sport beyond that of merely participating as a performer. *(2 marks)*

4 The government has set a number of school PE/sports targets, including a minimum of 2 hours' National Curriculum PE for each child per week by 2008. Why might some schools find it difficult to make this recommended provision for their students? *(3 marks)*

5 How can organisations such as NGBs try to achieve equality of opportunity and increase participation in sport for different social groups? *(4 marks)*

Chapter 13

Barriers to participation

What you need to know

By the end of this section you should be able to:
- understand key terms linked to equal opportunities in sport, including discrimination, stereotyping, prejudice and inclusiveness
- identify the barriers to participation for various target groups, including disability, socioeconomic class, ethnicity and gender
- suggest solutions to overcome discrimination in sport and raise participation

Key terms

Discrimination: unfair treatment of a person, racial group, minority; action based on prejudice.

Inclusive sport: where all people have the right to equal opportunities according to their particular needs.

Prejudice: to form an unfavourable opinion before meeting an individual, often based on inadequate facts, for example lack of tolerance of people from a specific race or religion.

Social exclusion: when certain sections of society are left out of the mainstream; this can happen when people suffer from a range of linked problems, for example unemployment, low income and poor housing.

Stereotyping: a set of simplistic generalisations about a group that allows others to categorise them and treat them accordingly.

Terminology

There are a number of key terms you need to understand when studying equal opportunities in sport and recreation. Three of these — prejudice, discrimination and stereotyping — are important reasons for inequality, both in the past and at present.

The lack of participation of the four groups identified in the Unit 1 specification — that is, women, ethnic minorities, the disabled and lower social classes — can be linked to a number of different factors, including prejudice, discrimination and stereotyping. Increasing participation in sport is helping to achieve an important aim for local and central government — to decrease exclusion (and therefore increase inclusion) in society. Local and national governments continue to invest resources in sport and recreation schemes to try to create a sense of value/worth in society in an effort to combat social exclusion.

The performance pyramid

A pyramid structure can be used to illustrate a continuum of development from mass participation at the base of the pyramid through to excellence at the top.

The performance pyramid has four levels. At the bottom is the **foundation** level, which is the first introduction to physical activity for young children, often during primary school PE. Basic movement skills and a positive attitude to physical activity are developed from an early age. It is sometimes referred to as the 'grass-roots' stage of development.

The second level is **participation**, with an emphasis on fun, socialising and formation of friendships in a recreational manner. At school this may be through extra-curricular activities.

More dedicated individuals may reach the **performance** stage. Such individuals reach county or regional levels of performance and receive specialist coaching in order to try to improve their standard. This stage is a focus of Unit 3.

A limited few reach **excellence** as elite performers. Such individuals strive to represent their country and are fully committed to their sport. In some cases they receive financial support to enable them to train full time and achieve success in international sporting competitions. This again is a focus of Unit 3 as it considers how the UK is developing its elite performers to compete more effectively on the world sporting stage.

Our focus in Unit 1 is on the bottom two levels of the pyramid. Our consideration of various target groups is concerned with widening the base of the pyramid at foundation level and increasing the numbers participating recreationally, that is, at the participation level.

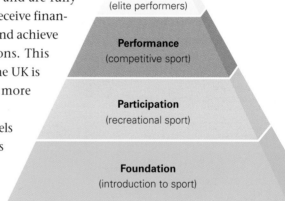

Figure 13.1 The performance pyramid

Sport and mass participation

The focus of Unit 1 is on how we can raise levels of participation at the bottom two levels of the performance pyramid, that is, how we can increase mass participation.

The idea behind mass participation in sport is that everyone should have the chance to take part as often as they would like and at whatever level they choose. However, reality does not always match the principle of equal opportunities in 'Sport for All'. Target and special interest groups are sections of society identified by Sport England as needing special attention. The aim is to raise participation levels to try to ensure that these groups have equality of sporting opportunity.

Examples of target groups include ethnic minorities, women, young people (16–24), the elderly, lower social-class groups and people with disabilities. They are of special interest due to their under-representation in physical activity in relation to their numbers in society.

> **Top tip**
>
> Make sure you can identify and explain the bottom two levels of the pyramid in your own words, as this may be asked for in an exam.

Sport for All is a UK policy, initiated in the 1970s, aimed at achieving mass participation. In reality, however, not everyone is able to take up the sport of his/her choice. Various constraints limit regular participation. These can be grouped under three main headings:

- **opportunity** — factors that affect the chance to take part in sport or recreation, including time, money and the attitudes of friends and family
- **provision** — more tangible features that affect participation, including the availability of specialist facilities, equipment, coaching and appropriate activities
- **self-esteem** — the self-confidence to take part and the effects of perceptions held by others of an individual or group. Self-esteem is affected by an individual's status in a stratified society. It can lead to low expectations and under-achievement among lower social classes, people with disabilities and ethnic minorities. For example, social class may affect money available for equipment, coaching and transport.

Combinations of factors can lead to double deprivation and a greater likelihood of under-representation. For example, if you are a woman with disabilities, you are less likely to participate than if you are a man with disabilities or if you are a woman without disabilities.

Under-representation of women in sport

Not all women want to perform in all activities. The key issue is when discrimination or gender stereotyping *denies* women the freedom to choose. Women should have the same opportunity as men both to participate and to excel in their chosen sport.

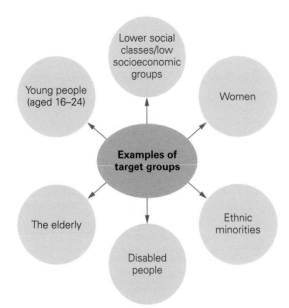

Figure 13.2 Examples of target groups

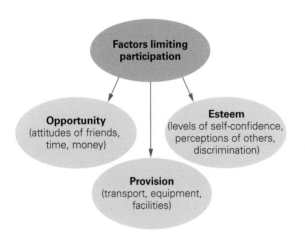

Figure 13.3 Factors limiting participation

Tasks to tackle 13.1

Consider your own experiences in sport and recreation and note any factors that have hindered your involvement in such physical activity.

A variety of different reasons can be given to explain the under-representation of women in sport. These include:

- stereotypical myths, for example the belief that physical activity could damage fertility, or that women are not aggressive
- less media coverage
- fewer role models and sponsorship opportunities
- lower prize money
- negative effects of school PE programmes, for example lack of choice, rules on kit
- lack of time due to work and family responsibilities
- lack of disposable income
- fewer female coaches and officials

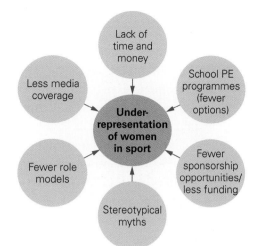

Figure 13.4 Under-representation of women in sport

Solutions to gender inequalities

Although women's representation in sport is still relatively low in relation to their numbers in society, improvements are being made. Reasons include the following:

- There is greater social acceptance of women having jobs and financial independence.
- Media coverage of women's sport has increased and positive role models have been promoted (e.g. Kelly Holmes).
- Stereotypical myths are refuted through education.
- More women are qualifying as coaches and to officiate in women's (and in some cases men's) sport.
- There are more clubs for women to join and more competitions to enter.
- Childcare is provided at some leisure centres.
- The Women's Sports Foundation (see **www.wsf.org.uk**) promotes the benefits of participation in exercise and female role models, and works with other organisations to develop campaigns and policies such as Sports Coach UK and Women into High Performance Coaching.

The Women's Sports Foundation has produced a fact sheet that illustrates why raising levels of participation in sport among women is important. It points out that sport:

- improves body image and self-esteem
- reduces stress and depression, and increases energy levels
- develops skills necessary for success in the workplace, for example strategic thinking, goal setting, teamwork
- lowers the risk of obesity and initiation of cigarette smoking in adolescent girls
- increases the chance of academic success
- increases the overall quality of life

Top tip

For case studies of initiatives in the UK that have worked to increase women's participation in physical activity, see www.whatworksforwomen.org.uk

Women's participation in indoor activities such as badminton and aerobics is relatively high compared with outdoor activities such as rugby and hockey. Reasons for this include:

- a comfortable environment (dry and warm)
- seen as good for health and fitness/body toning
- improved provision in school PE programmes and clubs (preparation for leisure)
- activities can be performed recreationally, as lifetime activities
- they are non-contact activities
- they are more socially acceptable and fit female stereotypes

However, it should be noted that association football is gaining in popularity among women. A number of sociocultural factors can help to explain this:

- increased equal opportunities in society in general
- increased media coverage of women's football, for example the women's World Cup in China, 2007

Top tip

Exam questions often require knowledge of causes of under-representation of women in sport and suggested solutions to these barriers. For example, if lack of time due to childcare responsibilities is a continuing barrier to participation, provision of crèches at leisure centres is one solution.

Top tip

Do some informal research on media coverage of women's sport by comparing a few newspapers to see how much coverage women get compared with men.

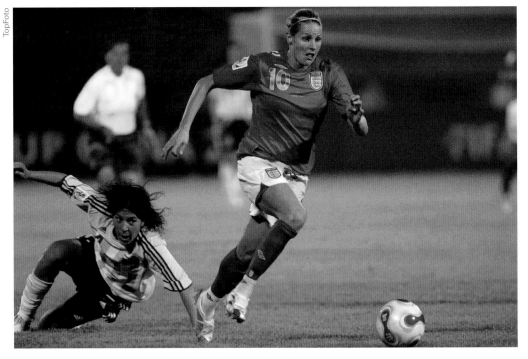

England versus Argentina in the 2007 FIFA Women's World Cup

- more female role models
- more opportunities for girls to play football in school PE programmes
- more clubs to join
- rejection of stereotypes affecting female participation in contact activities such as football
- more leisure time and disposable income available

Task to tackle 13.2

How might women be discriminated against in sport?

Race and religion in sport

Britain is a multicultural, multiracial egalitarian society. Equal opportunities to participate in sport should exist for all racial groups. Such equality is not a reality due to many factors, including racism.

Racism is illegal but it still exists in society (and therefore in sport as a reflection of society) on the basis of colour, language or culture. Racism stems from prejudice linked with the power of one racial group over another. This leads to discrimination, or unfair treatment. For example, teachers might assign students to certain sports or positions on the basis of ascribed ethnic characteristics rather than interests and abilities.

Other causes of under-representation of certain ethnic groups in sports and physical recreation include:

- conflict with religious observances
- a higher value placed on education (less support from family for sports participation)
- racist abuse
- fewer role models (particularly as coaches and managers)
- lower self-esteem and fear of rejection

Possible solutions to racial disadvantage and discrimination include:

- training more ethnic minority sports teachers and coaches, and educating them on the effects of stereotyping
- ensuring there is single-sex provision for Muslim women
- publicising and punishing more severely any racist abuse
- organising campaigns against racism in sport, for example the Kick It Out campaign
- making more provision in PE programmes for different ethnic preferences, for example by relaxing kit and showering rules to accommodate cultural norms

Ethnic groups: people who have racial, religious or linguistic traits in common.

Racism: a set of beliefs based on the assumption that races have distinct hereditary characteristics that give some races an intrinsic superiority over others. It may lead to physical or verbal abuse.

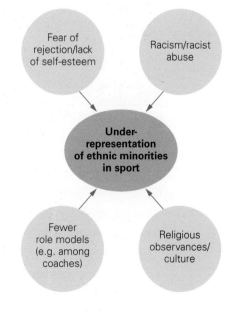

Figure 13.5 Barriers to participation for ethnic minority groups

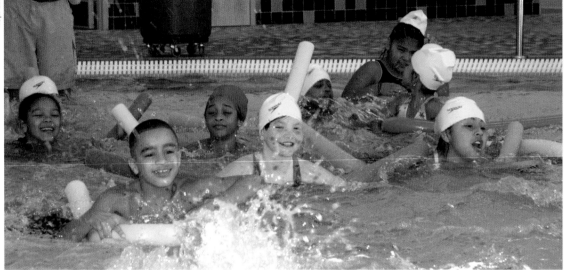

Equal opportunities in PE and sport need to take account of cultural differences

Under-representation of the disabled in sport

Generally, people with disabilities have a low level of participation in sport. Disability may be physical, sensory or mental in nature, with all of these potentially affecting participation in a negative way. Society continues to discriminate against, and impose barriers on, disabled people's participation in physical activity.

Reasons why individuals with disabilities do not participate in physical activity include:

- negative self-image — this often adversely affects the confidence to take part, particularly when reinforced by negative comments and reactions from the public
- lower income levels — three-quarters of disabled people rely on state benefits as their main source of income
- lack of appropriate transport and access into and around facilities
- lack of specialist coaches
- lack of specialist equipment to meet the needs of disabled people
- fewer competitive opportunities
- low levels of media coverage

For some disabled individuals, inclusiveness is best realised by integration, while for others segregation may be better.

Integration has potentially a number of benefits for disabled individuals, such as increasing their self-esteem, breaking down negative stereotypes and helping them feel more valued in society. However, integration can also affect people with disabilities in negative ways, including safety concerns that have to be addressed and lower self-esteem if they are continually unsuccessful.

Segregation may lead to positive outcomes for the disabled, such as increased success. The negative aspects of segregation include reinforcement of the notion that the disabled are different from the rest of society, which may make them feel less valued and excluded from mainstream society.

The Paralympic Games have had a positive impact on the involvement of disabled people in sport. Media coverage has raised the profile of disabled sport and educated the general public about how disabled athletes compete in various sports, for example through adaptations.

Disability Sport England (www.dse.org.uk) is a specialist organisation involved in trying to increase participation among people with disabilities. It has a number of important functions, including:

- promotion of the benefits of exercise to the disabled
- supporting relevant organisations who provide for the disabled in sport and recreation
- increasing awareness and knowledge in society of the needs and abilities of disabled individuals
- encouraging disabled individuals to play an active role in the development of their sport
- enhancing the image and understanding of disability sport

Benefits of participating in sport for disabled individuals include:

- raised levels of confidence and self-esteem
- improved levels of physical skill

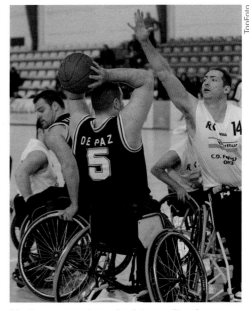
TopFoto

Media coverage has raised the profile of some disabled sports

Key terms

Inclusiveness: the idea that all people should have their needs, abilities and aspirations recognised, understood and met within a supportive environment.

Integration: able-bodied and disabled people taking part in the same activity at the same time.

Segregation: people with disabilities participating separately among themselves.

Table 13.1 Causes of, and solutions to, under-representation of disabled individuals in sport

Cause	Solution
Negative self-image, lack of confidence	Provide opportunities for success
Low income levels	Increase investment in disabled sport to make it more affordable
Poor access to facilities, poor access in and around them	Provide transport to facilities; improve access in and around them
Low levels of media coverage, few role models	Increase media coverage of disabled sport, e.g. the Paralympics
Low levels of funding	Increase funding from the National Lottery
Few competitions and clubs	More competitions at all levels; more clubs for the disabled in a wider variety of sports
Myths and stereotypes	Educate people about the myths concerning disabled individuals and challenge inappropriate attitudes

Chapter 13 — Barriers to participation

- increased health and fitness
- inclusion and integration into society
- more role models to encourage participation
- reducing myths and stereotypes about the disabled

Effects of social class

In Britain, social class, wealth discrimination and the consequent inequality of opportunity are centuries old. In pre-industrial times (early 1700s), the upper and lower social classes pursued separate sports. For example, hunting was exclusively for the upper classes and mob football was for the lower classes. As a result of the Industrial Revolution, a new middle class was created that participated in sport 'for the love of the game' and played a key role in the formation of the national governing bodies and subsequent rule development. A three-tier society is still broadly in evidence in the UK today and can be linked to sporting participation as follows:

- upper class — polo, equestrianism and field sports
- middle class — hockey, tennis, golf and rugby union
- working class — football, darts, snooker and rugby league

There is also evidence that lower socioeconomic background leads to less participation in sport. This is due to factors such as cost, lower levels of health and fitness, low self-esteem and lack of opportunities to take up sport or to become role models in positions of responsibility. People from lower socioeconomic backgrounds are more likely to suffer from social exclusion as they have less power, income and self-confidence — they suffer from a range of linked problems such as higher unemployment, lower income and poor health.

Subsidised provision that encourages participation in local community schemes can help to overcome these barriers; for example Sport Action Zones were set up by Sport England in some inner city areas. Such schemes also serve important functions as diversions from crime and general social disorder.

There are four clearly defined **Top tip** target groups you need to study — ethnic minority groups, women, people with disabilities and lower socioeconomic groups. You need to consider causes of lower levels of participation in sport and recreation and possible solutions to such problems.

Tasks to tackle 13.3

Discuss whether social class still affects participation in sport.

Practice makes perfect

1 Explain what is meant by **mass participation**. *(2 marks)*

2 What factors have led to an increase in the opportunities for women to participate in football in the UK? *(4 marks)*

3 Identify a range of different factors that can influence an individual's participation in sport and recreation. *(5 marks)*

Unit 2

Analysis and evaluation of physical activity as a performer and/or in adopted roles

Chapter *14*

Training and fitness testing

What you need to know

By the end of this chapter you should be able to:

- apply the principles of training and understand the concepts of specificity, progression, moderation (over-training), overload (FITT), reversibility and variance (tedium)
- calculate working intensities for optimal gains by heart rate, Borg scale and one rep max
- understand the reasons for testing, and know the principles of maximal and submaximal tests, the limitations of testing, specific test protocols and issues relating to validity and reliability
- understand the physiological and psychological value of a warm-up and cool-down, types of stretching exercise (active, passive, static and ballistic) and know the principles of safe practice
- explain the principles of various training methods — continuous, intermittent, circuit, weights, plyometrics and mobility training — and give examples, advantages and disadvantages of each method

Principles of training

Fitness can be improved by following an effective training programme that includes the six principles of training.

Overload (FITT)

Overload is achieved by increasing one or more of the following:

- **frequency** — the number of training sessions per week. This depends on the amount of time the individual can devote to training. It may be more convenient to increase the intensity or duration of an individual session.
- **intensity** — how hard the performer works. For example, it is possible to increase the intensity of a run by increasing the pace or by adding some uphill sections. To increase aerobic fitness, it is important to increase the intensity of the exercise by training above the aerobic threshold but below the anaerobic threshold. Training zones help us to do this. They are discussed on pp. 149–50.
- **time** — the duration of the session. Overloading will require an increase in time, for example a 30-minute run could increase to a 40-minute run. Whatever the increase in time, each session should last a minimum of 20 minutes.

- **type** — the type of training that is most suitable for what you want to achieve. For example, to increase stamina (cardio-respiratory endurance), continuous training is one type that can help to achieve this.

Progression

Progression involves the gradual application of overload. It is important to overload the body in order to improve fitness but this should be done progressively.

Specificity

Specificity involves keeping the training relevant. For example, a sprinter will do strength training on the muscles required for his/her event and speed training to improve the efficiency of the energy system used when competing.

Reversibility

Reversibility is often referred to as detraining. If training stops, the adaptations that have occurred as a result of training deteriorate. It has been suggested that aerobic adaptations are lost more quickly than strength adaptations.

Moderation (over-training)

Moderation — don't overdo it! Over-training can lead to injury.

Variance (tedium)

A training programme needs to have variety in order to maintain interest and motivation.

Calculating working intensities for optimal gains

Heart rate

Heart rate training zones can be used to gauge how hard you are working. Most training zones are calculated from the maximum heart rate. An estimate of maximum heart rate is calculated as:

220 – your age

So if you are 17, your maximum heart rate is calculated as:

220 – 17 = 203

You then need to work at a certain percentage of this maximum heart rate. One way of doing this is to use the Karvonen principle. The Karvonen principle is more accurate than other methods because it takes into account individual fitness levels. Resting heart rate is used to work out an individual's training zone. Karvonen suggests a training intensity of 60–75% of maximum heart rate, using the following calculation:

60% = resting heart rate (+ 0.6 × (max. heart rate − resting heart rate))

75% = resting heart rate + 0.75 × (max. heart rate − resting heart rate)

For a 17-year-old with a resting heart rate of 60 beats per minute, the calculation is:

60% = 60 + 0.6 (203 − 60)   75% = 70 + 0.75 (203 − 60)
     = 60 + 0.6 × 143   = 70 + 0.75 × 143
     = 60 + 86 (85.8)   = 70 + 107 (107.25)
     = 146   = 177

Therefore, a 17-year-old with a resting heart rate of 60, working at an intensity of 60–75% of maximum heart rate, should be working with a heart rate of between 146 and 177 beats per minute.

Borg scale

The Borg scale is a simple method of rating perceived exertion (RPE) and is used to measure a performer's level of intensity during training. Perceived exertion is how hard you feel your body is working. During exercise, the Borg scale is used to assign numbers to how you feel. If you feel you are working too hard, you can reduce the intensity. There are numerous RPE scales but the most common ones are the 15-point scale and the 9-point scale. The 15-point scale is illustrated in Figure 14.1.

Key term

Perceived exertion: how hard you feel your body is working during exercise.

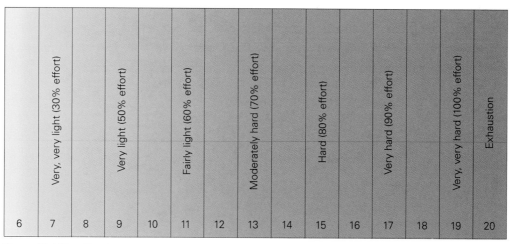

Figure 14.1 The 15-point perceived exertion scale

One rep max

When weight training you need to work out your one repetition maximum (1RM) for each exercise that you plan to do, so that you can decide on the intensity that you want to train at.

There are different types of strength and you need to decide which type you want to improve. Depending on strength type, you need to work at a certain percentage of your 1RM. For example:

- maximum strength: 85% and over of 1RM
- power (elastic strength): 70–85% of 1RM
- muscular endurance: 50–70% of 1RM

The heavier the weights, the fewer repetitions you will be able to do. For example, for maximum strength, working at 85% would need about 4–5 sets with 6 repetitions, but 95% would be 3–4 sets with 2–4 reps.

Training methods

Continuous training

Continuous training concentrates on developing endurance, which places stress on the aerobic energy system. It involves exercise without rest intervals. Examples include exercises such as cycling, jogging and swimming.

In order to gain any improvement in aerobic fitness, it is important to follow the principles of training:

- Frequency — training must take place at least two or three times per week.
- Intensity — this should be at about 60–75% of maximum heart rate.
- Time — the training session should last at least 20 minutes, but ideally between 30 minutes and 2 hours to ensure the aerobic system is working fully.
- Progression — after a few weeks the body will adapt to the exercise, so resting heart rate is reduced. Therefore, to ensure you are working at 60–75% of maximum heart rate, you will have to work harder by increasing frequency, intensity or time.
- Specificity — the training session should be specific to the requirements of the activity. It has been suggested that training should be over a distance of between two and five times that covered in the activity.
- Moderation — don't overdo it.
- Variance — keep training sessions interesting. Vary the loads, skills and activities.
- Reversibility — the aerobic fitness level will drop if training stops.

Fartlek training

The word 'fartlek' is Swedish and means speed-play. This is a slightly different method of continuous training where the pace of the run is varied to stress both the aerobic and the anaerobic energy systems. This is a much more demanding type of training, which improves VO_2 (max) and the recovery process. A typical session lasts for about 40 minutes, with the intensity ranging from low to high.

The individual determines the intensity and duration of training. Fartlek training offers more variety through the use of both aerobic and anaerobic work and is beneficial to games players where the demands of the game are constantly changing, so that both types of respiration are required.

A typical fartlek session involves varying the pace of a run by integrating sprints into the workout, and following these with recovery runs in the form of slow jogs. The route can also be varied to include both uphill and downhill work. For example:

- 10 minutes jogging
- 6 × (20 seconds fast running with 80 seconds recovery)
- 5 minutes walk
- 5 minutes jog
- 2 × (run uphill for 1 minute, jog down)
- 3 minutes jogging
- 2 minutes walking

Intermittent (interval) training

Intermittent training is particularly popular with elite athletes. It is used most frequently in athletics, cycling and swimming and can improve both aerobic and anaerobic capacities. In intermittent training, periods of work are interspersed with recovery periods. Four main variables are used to ensure the training is specific:

- the duration of the work interval
- the intensity or speed of the work interval
- the duration of the recovery period
- the number of work intervals and recovery periods

It is possible to adapt interval training to overload each of the three energy systems (see Table 14.1). ATP–PC intervals have to be short and high intensity, for example at 90–100% of maximum effort. This allows for increases in muscle stores of ATP and phosphocreatine. Lactic acid intervals need to be moderate to high intensity, lasting between 15 and 90 seconds. This is so that the athlete can train with some lactic acid present in order to improve the buffering capacity of the blood. Aerobic intervals are much longer (up to 10 minutes duration) and at lower intensity. This improves the oxidative capacity of the body.

Table 14.1 Intermittent training

Energy system	Duration/distance of work interval	Intensity of work interval	Duration of recovery	Number of work intervals/recovery periods
ATP–PC	10 s /60 m	High	30 s	10
Lactic acid	35 s/200 m	High	110 s	8
Aerobic	6 min/1500 m	Submaximal	5 min	3

The advantage of intermittent training is that it can be adapted to suit almost anyone, from the sprinter to the endurance athlete to the games player. A 100 metres sprinter will want to improve his/her ATP–PC system. A 400 metres sprinter will concentrate on the lactic acid system. Endurance athletes will seek improvements to their aerobic system.

The three energy systems are studied in more detail at A2.

Strength training

Some individuals do a form of strength training to improve performance in their chosen activity. Improvements in strength result from working against some form of resistance. In this instance, it is also important to make any strength-training programme specific to the needs of the activity. To do this, the following factors must be considered:

- the type of strength to be developed — maximum, elastic (power) or muscular endurance
- the muscle groups to be improved
- the type of muscle contraction performed in the activity — concentric, eccentric or isometric

Other individuals do strength training for muscle growth. They need to ensure that any exercises they perform will overload the anaerobic energy systems, which will result in hypertrophy of fast-twitch fibres.

Strength can be improved by doing the following types of training:

- weights — high weights for maximum and elastic strength, low weights for muscular endurance
- circuits for muscular endurance
- plyometrics and pulleys for elastic strength

Strength training is important to avoid muscle loss that occurs with ageing. It can help to increase physical capacity, improve athletic performance and reduce the risk of injury.

Weight training

Weight training involves doing a series of resistance exercises designed to develop the fitness component for particular sport-related muscles. The exercises are usually described in terms of sets and repetitions. The number of sets and repetitions and the amount of weight lifted depend on the type of strength to be improved.

Before a programme can be designed, it is important to determine the maximum amount of weight that the performer can lift with one repetition (1RM). Then, if maximum strength is the goal, it will be necessary to lift high weights with low repetitions, for example, 2–6 repetitions at 80–100% of maximum strength. However if muscular endurance is the goal, it will be necessary to perform more repetitions of lighter weights, for example, three sets of 10 repetitions at approximately 50% of maximum strength.

The choice of exercise should relate to the muscle groups used in sport — both the agonists and antagonists. The exercises are usually classed in four groups:

- shoulders and arms, for example bench press, curls, pull downs
- trunk and back, for example sit-ups, back hyperextensions

- legs, for example squats, calf raises, leg press
- whole body exercises, for example power clean, snatch, dead lift

Circuit training

In circuit training, the athlete performs a series of exercises in succession. These exercises should include arm exercises such as press-ups and triceps dips, leg exercises such as squat thrusts, and trunk exercises such as sit-ups and dorsal raises, as well as cardiovascular exercises such as jogging and skipping.

The resistance used is the athlete's body weight and each exercise concentrates on a different muscle group to allow for recovery. A circuit is usually designed for general body conditioning and it is easily adapted to meet the needs of an activity. An example of a circuit is shown in Figure 14.2.

A circuit is usually designed for general body conditioning but can be easily adapted to include skill training.

Most circuits involve the performer working for a period of between 30 seconds and 1 minute, with a similar recovery period. The recovery period is usually active — jogging or walking.

Most circuits are completed in pairs, with one person recovering while the other works.

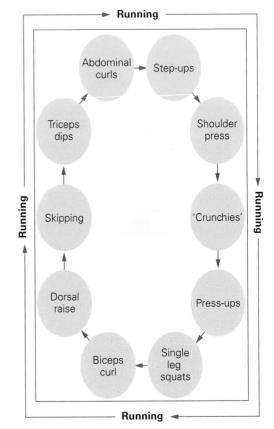

Figure 14.2 A typical circuit for circuit training

Plyometrics

If leg strength is crucial to successful performance, for example in the long jump and the 100 m sprint in athletics, or rebounding in basketball, then plyometrics is one method of strength training that can be used to improve power or elastic strength.

Plyometrics works on the concept that muscles can generate more force if they have previously been stretched. This occurs in plyometrics when, on landing, the muscle performs an eccentric contraction (lengthens under tension) followed immediately by a concentric contraction as the performer jumps up. This stimulates adaptations within the neuromuscular system and results in a more powerful concentric contraction of the muscle group being worked.

For example, to develop leg strength, a line of benches, boxes and hurdles is made and the performer has to jump, hop and leap from one to the other. Recovery occurs during the walk back to the start line and the exercise is repeated.

Arm strength can be developed by performing press-ups with mid-air claps, or by throwing and catching a medicine ball.

Strength gains through plyometrics usually become apparent following a training period of about 8–10 weeks. This is due to muscle hypertrophy (an increase in the size of the muscle).

Mobility (flexibility) training

Mobility training involves stretching the muscles and connective tissue. A stretch should be held for at least 10 seconds and a session should last for 10 minutes. With regular and repeated stretching, this soft tissue can elongate and this may be beneficial in avoiding injury.

There are three main types of flexibility training:

- static stretching
- ballistic stretching
- PNF

Static stretching can be active or passive. In active stretching, the performer works on one joint, pushing it beyond its point of resistance, lengthening the muscles and connective tissue surrounding it. In passive stretching, the stretch occurs with the help of an external force, such as a partner, gravity or a wall.

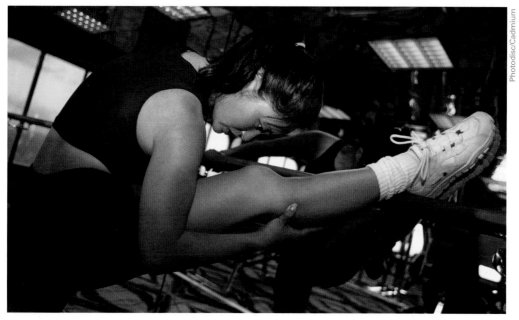

A stretch should be held for at least 10 seconds

Ballistic stretching involves performing a stretch with swinging or bouncing movements to push a body part even further. Only individuals who are extremely flexible, such as gymnasts and dancers, should perform this type of stretching.

PNF (proprioceptive neuromuscular facilitation) is where the muscle is contracted isometrically for a period of at least 10 seconds. It then relaxes and is stretched again, usually going further the second time.

Fitness testing

There are tests for each type of fitness. Fitness testing measures a performer's ability and is beneficial to both the performer and the coach in highlighting areas for improvement. Fitness testing can:

- highlight strengths and weaknesses
- allow progress to be monitored carefully, through re-testing and comparison to norms
- help to motivate an individual if improvements are made
- monitor the success of a training programme — if no improvement is seen, the training programme can be modified
- help in talent identification

Principles of maximal and submaximal tests

Maximal tests are performed when the athlete is working at maximum effort, usually to exhaustion. The tests are reliable and objective. Examples of anaerobic maximal tests are the 30 m sprint and the Wingate test (see p. 158). Aerobic maximal tests include the multistage fitness test and Cooper's 12-minute run (see p. 157).

Disadvantages of these types of test are as follows:

- It is difficult to ensure that the performer is actually working to a maximum.
- It is hard to stay motivated when pushing yourself to exhaustion.
- There are possible dangers of over-exertion and injury.

Submaximal tests are not exhaustive and do not require the performer to work at maximal levels. Aerobic examples of these tests include the Harvard step test and the PWC170 test. Motivation is no longer an issue. However, these tests rely on data that are predictive or estimated, and there are problems with accuracy and objectivity.

Validity and reliability of testing

The two main issues to consider in fitness testing are validity and reliability. Validity relates to whether the test actually measures what it sets out to measure. For example, the sit-and-reach test assesses flexibility but only covers the hamstrings and the lower back. It is therefore a valid test for the lower body but not for the upper body.

It is important to conduct a test so that it replicates the sporting actions and uses the muscles in the same way as the performer uses them during the activity. For example, the multistage fitness test involves running, so it is a valid for a games player where a lot of running is involved but is less valid for a cyclist or a swimmer.

Reliability is a question of whether the test is accurate. For example, for the step test to be reliable, it is important to ensure that the procedure is correctly maintained. This means that everyone who completes the test does so at the same rate and step height, and that there is full extension between steps.

The following factors must be taken into account when testing:

- The tester should be experienced.
- Equipment should be standardised.
- The sequencing of tests is important. For example, it is not a good idea to do two maximal tests, such as the multistage fitness test (see below) and the NCF abdominal curl test (see p. 159), together.
- Different performers might have differing motivation to complete the test to the best of their ability.
- Tests should be repeated to avoid human error.

Evaluation of stamina

The various methods of evaluating stamina (cardio-respiratory endurance) include:

- the multistage fitness test
- Cooper's 12-minute run
- the Harvard step test
- the PWC170 cycle ergometer test

The multistage fitness test was developed by the National Coaching Foundation. The athlete performs a 20m progressive shuttle run in time with a beep, to the point of exhaustion. The level reached depends on the number of shuttle runs completed and is ascertained from a standard results table. The testing procedure is simple, and it provides a guide to measure progress. Large groups of people can be tested together, so it is not time consuming. However, it only gives an estimate of VO$_2$ max. It is a maximal test and involves running, so it is of little relevance to, say, swimmers.

Table 14.2 VO$_2$ max averages/ml kg^{-1} min^{-1}

Females aged 18–25	Males aged 18–25	Rating
>56	>60	Excellent
47–56	52–60	Good
42–46	47–51	Above average
38–41	42–46	Average
33–37	37–41	Below average
28–32	30–36	Poor
<28	<30	Very poor

Cooper's 12-minute run requires the athlete to run as far as he/she can in 12 minutes. The testing procedure is simple and very little equipment is needed. Large groups can be tested together and standardised data are used for comparison. This, too, is a maximal test.

The Harvard step test involves the athlete stepping up and down rhythmically on a bench for 5 minutes. The recovery heart rate is then measured. The testing procedure is simple and the test is submaximal. The results depend on manual recording of the heart rate, which could lead to errors. Some participants will have difficulty keeping to the stepping rate, and stepping is not sport specific.

The PWC170 test involves three consecutive 4-minute workloads on a cycle ergometer. Each workload has a target heart rate: (1) 115–130, (2) 130–145, (3) 145–165. The heart rate for each workload is plotted on a graph and a line of best fit is drawn. This is a submaximal test and the weight of the performer is supported by the saddle. However, cycling is not relevant to many sports, and human error is possible in recording the heart rate, plotting the graph and drawing the line of best fit.

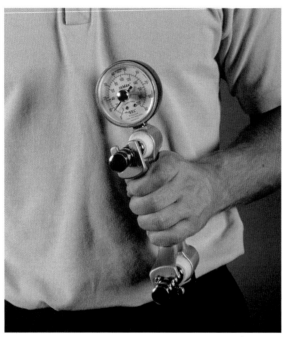

Handgrip dynamometer

Evaluation of strength

One simple method of assessing maximum strength is the handgrip test, using a muscle dynamometer. The performer squeezes the dynamometer while lowering it from shoulder height to the side. The highest reading from three attempts is recorded. The testing procedure is straight-forward but the test concentrates on the muscular strength of the forearm and is therefore limited.

Table 14.3 Handgrip dynamometer ratings/kg

Males	Females	Rating
>65	>36	Excellent
50–65	31–36	Good
40–49	25–30	Average
30–39	19–24	Fair
<30	<19	Poor

The 1RM test requires the performer to lift the maximum weight he/she can, just once. Trial and error is needed to find this maximum so ample rest should be allowed between attempts. The procedure is simple, all muscle groups can be tested and the test can be sport specific. However, access to a multigym is needed and there is a risk of injury.

Power (elastic strength) can be assessed under laboratory conditions by the Wingate test. The resistance on a cycle ergometer is adjusted according to body weight — 75 g per kilogram of body weight. Maximum effort is required for a period of over 30 s. The number of pedal revolutions is counted every 5 s of the test. The test yields objective data but it is a maximal test requiring expensive equipment and is sport specific for cyclists only.

The vertical jump test is a simpler method of assessing power. The performer's standing reach is measured against a wall. He/she then jumps and reaches as high as possible from a squatting position and the height is recorded. Different techniques are used (for example, standing sideways on or facing the wall, slapping the wall or sliding the arm up the wall), so there is a lack of consistency. In addition, it is difficult to time the jump so that a mark can be made when the performer is at full height.

A test for muscular endurance assesses the ability of one or more muscle groups to work continuously. The NCF abdominal curl test measures the endurance of the abdominal muscles. The test involves doing sit-ups in time with a beat until complete exhaustion is reached. The testing procedure is simple and large groups of people can be tested together. It is a maximal test. Care must be taken to use the correct technique because a lot of strain can be placed on the lumbar region of the spine.

Flexibility

The sit-and-reach test gives an indication of flexibility of the hamstrings and lower back. To complete the test, a sit-and-reach box is required. The performer sits on the floor with feet flat against the box, legs straight. Slowly he/she reaches forward as far as possible, pushing the marker with the fingertips. This position must be held for a couple of seconds. The score is read and compared with a rating from tabulated values. This is an easy test to set up and perform but it tests only the hamstrings and lower back.

Coordination

An easy self-evaluation test is the alternate-hand wall toss. The performer stands 2 metres from a wall with a tennis ball in her right hand. She throws the ball underarm against the wall and catches it with her left

Table 14.4 Vertical jump test ratings

Height jumped/cm, males	Height jumped/cm, females	Rating
>59	>46	Excellent
51–59	36–46	Good
41–50	29–35	Average
<41	<29	Poor

Table 14.5 NCF abdominal curl test ratings

Stage	Number of sit-ups (cumulative)	Rating	
		Male	Female
1	20	Poor	Poor
2	42	Poor	Fair
3	64	Fair	Fair
4	89	Fair	Good
5	116	Good	Good
6	146	Good	Very good
7	180	Excellent	Excellent
8	217	Excellent	Excellent

Table 14.6 Sit-and-reach test ratings/cm

Male	Female	Rating
>34	>38	Excellent
31–34	33–38	Good
27–30	29–32	Fair
<27	<29	Poor

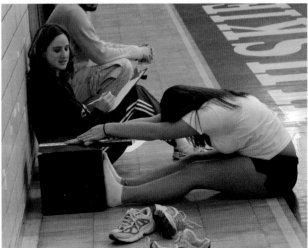

Dennis MacDonald/Alamy

Students assessing flexibility using the sit-and-reach test

hand. Then she throws the ball from her left hand and catches it with the right. The number of successful catches made in 30 seconds is recorded. There is no rating for this test but a retest can be done at a later date to check for improvement. A drawback of this test is that it is not sport specific.

Speed

In the 30 metre sprint test the performer runs 30 m as fast as he/she can. The time is compared with a rating table. Limitations of the test include: possible human error in the timing, the result may be affected by the running surface and by the weather; and it is not sport specific because there is no change in direction.

Balance

The stork stand is a test used to evaluate static balance. The performer stands with hands on hips, lifts one foot and rests it on the knee of the other leg. The heel of the straight leg is then raised so that the performer is balancing on his/her toes. The balance is held for as long as possible and the time is recorded. The results can be compared with standardised data. The main limitation of the stork stand is that it is a static balance test. It is not sport specific and most activities require dynamic balance.

Table 14.7 Alternate-hand wall toss ratings

Number of throws in 30 s	Rating
>35	Excellent
30–35	Good
20–29	Average
15–19	Fair
<15	Poor

Table 14.8 30 metre sprint ratings/s

Males	Females	Rating
<4	<4.5	Excellent
4–4.2	4.5–4.6	Good
4.3–4.4	4.7–4.8	Average
4.5–4.6	4.9–5	Fair
>4.6	>5	Poor

Table 14.9 Stork stand ratings/s

Time balance held	Rating
>50	Excellent
40–50	Good
26–39	Average
11–25	Below average
<11	Poor

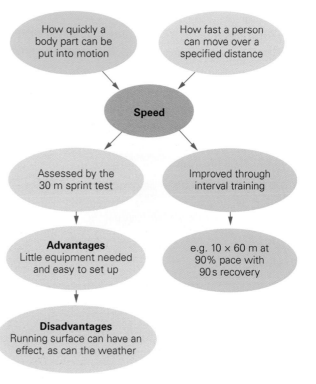

Figure 14.3 Assessing and improving

Agility

Agility is assessed by the Illinois agility run. The performer runs around a 10 m course as fast as he/she can, weaving and sprinting between a series of four evenly spaced cones. The run is timed and rated by standard tables.

Drawbacks include the result being affected by the surface and weather conditions and that it is not sport specific.

Table 14.10 Illinois agility run ratings/s

Males	Females	Rating
<15.3	<17	Excellent
15.3–16	17–17.9	Good
16.1–18	18–21.7	Average
18.1–19	21.8–23	Fair
>19	>23	Poor

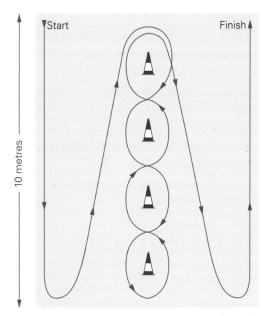

Figure 14.4 The Illinois agility run

Reaction time

A simple, cheap method of evaluating reaction time is the metre ruler test. A partner holds a metre ruler at the zero end. The performer places the index finger and thumb of his preferred hand on either side of the 50 cm mark, but not touching it. Without warning the partner lets go of the ruler and the performer must close his finger and thumb to catch it as close to the 50 cm mark as possible. The results can be compared with a rating table.

Table 14.11 Metre ruler test ratings

Reaction reading/cm	Rating
>42.4	Excellent
37–42.4	Good
29–36.9	Average
22–28.9	Fair
<22	Poor

Warming up and cooling down

The warm-up

A warm-up has both physiological and psychological benefits. It helps prepare the body for exercise and should always be carried out before the start of any training session.

The first stage of any warm-up is to perform some kind of cardiovascular exercise, such as jogging, gently increasing the pulse. This increases cardiac output and breathing rate and, through the vascular shunt, directs more blood to the working muscles.

The second stage is the performance of stretching and flexibility exercises, especially with those joints and muscles that will be most active during the training session.

The third stage should involve the movement patterns that are to be carried out, for example practising shooting in basketball and netball, or dribbling in hockey and football.

Together these three stages increase the amount of oxygen being delivered to the muscles and at the same time reduce the risk of injury.

A warm-up has the following physiological effects:

- The release of adrenaline increases heart rate and dilates the capillaries, allowing more oxygen to be delivered to the skeletal muscles.
- Muscle temperature increases, which enables oxygen to dissociate more easily from haemoglobin and allows for an increase in enzyme activity, making energy readily available.
- The speed of nerve impulse conduction increases, which increases alertness.
- The increase in muscle temperature leads to an increase in elasticity of the muscle fibres, which increases the speed and force of muscle contraction.
- Efficient movement at joints occurs through an increased production of synovial fluid.

The cool-down

After a heavy training session or a hard competitive match, there is a strong temptation to sit down and rest. However, it is important to perform a cool-down at the end of any physical activity as it helps to return the body to its pre-exercise state more quickly. Too many of us do not take the time to cool down properly.

A cool-down consists of some form of light exercise to keep the heart rate elevated. This keeps blood flow high and allows oxygen to be flushed through the muscles, oxidising and removing any lactic acid that remains.

Performing light exercise also allows the skeletal muscle pump to keep working and prevents blood from pooling in the veins. If we stop exercising suddenly, the amount of blood going back to the heart drops dramatically. This is because there is little or no muscle action to maintain the skeletal muscle pump. Consequently, stroke volume drops and there is a reduction in blood pressure. The performer will begin to feel dizzy and light-headed.

If an individual wants to improve strength, he/she will often work at higher intensities to overload the muscle in order to stimulate muscle hypertrophy. When this occurs, the individual may experience tender and painful muscles some 24–48 hours after exercise. This is called DOMS, or delayed onset of muscle soreness.

This muscle soreness results from the structural damage to muscle fibres and connective tissue surrounding the fibres. DOMS usually occurs following excessive eccentric contraction when muscle fibres are put under a lot of strain. This type of muscular contraction occurs mostly from weight training and plyometrics.

A thorough cool-down may help to limit the effect of DOMS.

Principles of safe practice

Apart from warming up and cooling down to help prevent injury and muscle soreness following exercise, there are some other factors that need to be considered:

- What exercises are to be done and in what order? It is important in circuits, for example, that muscle groups are rotated.

- Performers should always drink plenty of water during exercise to avoid dehydration.
- Rest days or recovery periods should be included in training sessions.
- The correct techniques must be used, especially in stretching and weight training.
- The safety of any equipment used must be checked. In weightlifting, for example, the collars on the bar must be tightened.
- Athletes training in a cold environment should wear plenty of layers of clothing.
- The sports hall should be clean and free from any potential dangers.
- Differences in performance due to gender and age should be considered. Generally, men have more strength than women but the opposite can be true for flexibility.
- Training should be progressive, whether you are fully fit or returning from injury.

Practice makes perfect

1 Describe a test used to measure flexibility. *(2 marks)*

2 What are the effects of a cool-down? *(2 marks)*

3 What are the advantages of intermittent training? *(2 marks)*

Chapter 15

Teaching and practice of skills

What you need to know

By the end of this chapter you should be able to:
- discuss the factors that need to be considered before a skill is taught
- understand the different practice and teaching methods available to a sports coach
- suggest when and how a coach could use those practice methods
- suggest advantages and disadvantages of those practice methods

In this section of the AQA specification you are asked to relate your theoretical knowledge to practical situations. In Section B of the exam paper you will be asked a question on the topics covered in this chapter. All the topics have been explained using practical examples to help you get the idea.

Coaching sports skills

The students' learning environment can be enhanced if the coach or teacher takes into account the factors that affect learning in sport and the classification of the skill. The planning of coaching sessions is important for effective learning and should take into account the nature of the task and the characteristics of the students being coached.

In terms of the nature of the task, the coach must be aware of the appropriate skills classification. If the skill is open, practice that takes into account the varied and changing nature of the skill should be undertaken. If the skill is closed, then practice could be repetitive. During the execution of an externally paced skill, the coach may want to place the performer under a little pressure so that he/she has to adapt. A self-paced skill can be executed in the player's own time. A gross skill may require contact and therefore a safety element to practice, while a fine skill may be performed in a calmer environment. Highly organised and discrete skills are more difficult to break down and may have to be practised in their entirety. Low-organised and serial tasks may be more easily broken down and can be practised in parts.

The coach must be aware of the characteristics of the students. If the students are well motivated and fit, a hard practice session with limited breaks could ensue. If the students are beginners, the coach may want to slow down the rate of practice and use rest intervals to emphasise certain points. The students' abilities should also be considered — it is no good doing complicated passing drills with students who have little coordination.

Teaching styles

The coach can choose to adopt one of three teaching styles:

- the command style
- the reciprocal style
- the problem-solving or discovery style

A coach who makes all the decisions and adopts an authoritarian approach uses the **command style**. This style is best used when there is danger — for example, telling a class of children not to dive into the shallow end of the swimming pool. The command style is good for large groups, because tight control can be maintained, and it is appropriate in situations where there is only one way of doing a task. It is an efficient method of teaching and is therefore useful when the coach has little time or is meeting deadlines.

Learning is effective because the correct action is learned with concise instructions. However, a problem with the command style is that it does not cater for different abilities. A performer who is unable to do the set task might lose motivation and feel inferior, while someone who can extend the task beyond what is asked of them could also feel demotivated. No interaction between members of the group is allowed in this style. There is no creativity and the success of learning depends on the teacher, who must have tight control.

The **reciprocal style** of teaching is used when there is a mix of abilities within a group and the teacher decides to set the tasks for the lesson and hand over part of the teaching to the more able performers. For example, in a swimming lesson when the coach is unable to enter the water, he/she may ask expert swimmers to demonstrate starts and turns.

This style promotes communication and interaction within the group. It may generate new ideas for the coach and aid personal development of the more able performers, who gain both confidence and coaching experience. It also gives immediate feedback to the group. However, the reciprocal approach is time-consuming, and there is a danger that even the more able pupils may lack coaching skills and present incorrect information to the others.

The **problem-solving** or **discovery style** of teaching is used when the teacher sets a task for the performers to complete in their own way. For example, a gym coach may ask a group to work out ways of travelling across a mat.

This style promotes group interaction and allows performers to work at their own level, so that they can either extend their skills to more complex moves or complete the task in a simple way. All levels of performer are therefore allowed to succeed and should gain motivation and satisfaction.

Key terms

Command style: the teacher makes all the decisions — didactic learning.

Problem-solving or **discovery style:** the teacher lets the learners work out solutions in their own way.

Reciprocal style: the teacher hands over part of the teaching to other members of the group.

Tasks to tackle 15.1

Make a checklist of issues to consider before coaching a skill. Use the headings 'Task' and 'Performer'.

Top tip

Sometimes questions are very specific and ask you to discuss issues concerning *the task* that you might consider before coaching a skill. Make sure you don't mention the *performer*.

Distributed practice: allowing rest intervals between practice sessions.

Fixed practice: repetition of a drill.

Massed practice: training sessions with no rest interval.

Part practice: the skill is divided into subroutines in order to focus on specific cues during practice.

Varied practice: using different drills and methods in training sessions.

Whole practice: skills are practised in their entirety, with subroutines intact.

However, the problem-solving style is time-consuming and, without teacher control, incorrect results may be achieved and dangerous techniques could be developed.

Types of practice

The types of practice that the coach can choose to use are:

- whole practice
- whole–part–whole practice
- pure part practice
- progressive part practice
- massed practice
- distributed practice
- fixed practice
- varied practice

Whole practice

Whole practice means that the skill is performed in its entirety, with all its subroutines. Whole practice promotes fluency and understanding because the links between each subroutine are established. For example, in a tennis serve the toss of the ball and the timing of the strike must be coordinated.

Whole practice is used when the skill is:

- highly organised and cannot be broken down into its parts
- discrete, with a clear beginning and end
- simple and the information can easily be recalled

The coach chooses this type of practice to enable the performer to develop a feel for the whole task and to provide a more realistic method of practice. Consistency in the execution of the skill is achieved, so that the image of the skill is stored in the memory as a motor programme.

The problem with whole practice is that it may require learners to undertake a task that is

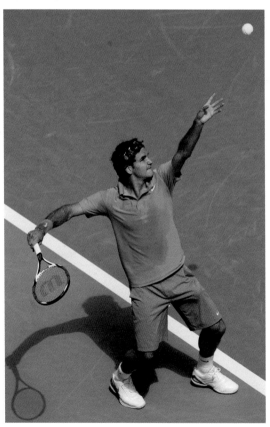

TopFoto

The subroutines of the tennis serve need to be coordinated during whole practice too advanced for them, with too much information for them to process at once.

Whole–part–whole practice

Whole–part–whole practice can be used to highlight a weakness in performance, or when a beginner is performing a complex task, or a task that is hard to break down. The task is performed in its entirety and the weaknesses are identified. The weaker parts are practised separately and are then integrated back into the whole task.

The whole–part–whole method of practice is useful when there is a particular point in technique that needs improvement and the skill is fluent and fast. For example, a particular point in the technique of a golf swing could be improved by focusing on one aspect before integrating this aspect back into the whole task.

Although it is time-consuming, this method is good for error correction, especially if the athlete is a more advanced performer.

Part methods of practice

Part practice is when a skill is split into subroutines and each part is practised separately. The parts are then reassembled to make the whole skill. Part practice is used when the skill is low in its organisation. There are two types of part practice:

- pure
- progressive

Pure part practice can be used when a skill is easily broken down into its subroutines. For example, a swimming stroke can be broken down into the leg action, the arm action, body position and breathing. Each of these can be practised independently.

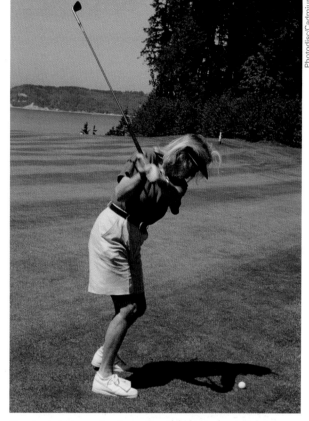

Fine tuning elements of a golf swing can be carried out in whole–part–whole practice

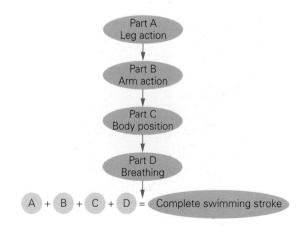

Figure 15.1 Learning a swimming stroke by the pure part method

Pure part practice is good for beginners, as it means that they are not given too much information at once and can concentrate on improving one aspect of the task at a time.

This method is also advantageous when there is an element of danger. By focusing on only part of the skill, the danger might be eliminated. For example, a trampolinist has to learn to do a basic move before trying something more complicated.

The disadvantages of pure part practice are that it is time-consuming and essential links between each subroutine of the skill may be neglected. For example, in breaststroke there is a link between the end of the leg kick and the start of the arm pull, called the glide phase. In pure part practice, this link may be neglected.

Progressive part practice attempts to solve one of the problems associated with pure part practice by maintaining the links between subroutines. The individual component parts of the task are practised separately and in the correct order, but at each stage the tasks are progressively linked to promote a fluid performance. Gradual progress is made.

Progressive part practice can be used:

- for serial skills in which each discrete element can be added in turn — for example, a dancer can add successive elements to complete a routine in this manner
- for beginners, so that they can make gradual progress
- for skills that are complex, so that the performer can concentrate on one part of the task at a time
- to reduce dangerous elements of a skill — by learning the early parts of the task before attempting the more difficult parts, risks are eliminated

For example, in the development of a dance routine the dancer might begin with the first two parts of the routine, say the turn and the kick, and practise these together. The third part of the skill, the leap, can be added to the routine later. The remaining parts of the sequence can be added until the whole routine is completed.

The drawbacks of progressive part practice are that it is time-consuming and there may be negative transfer between each part of the skill as it is learned.

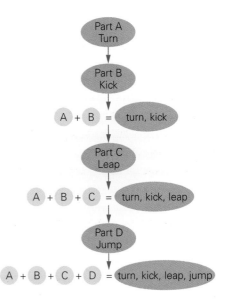

Figure 15.2 Learning a dance routine using the progressive part method

Massed practice

Massed practice is when no rest intervals are given between each component of the training session. It is used when a coach wants to promote a high level of fitness.

Massed practice has the advantage of promoting over-learning, so that the performer can cope with the demands of a real game. In rugby, for example, a coach who has put the players through their paces for an hour without a break, perhaps doing a pre-planned, structured routine, can be confident that they will cope with a 40-minute half game play.

This form of practice is appropriate for:

- simple skills that demand little attention, so the performer can still focus on the task after numerous attempts
- discrete skills with a clear end. These are usually short and sharp and can be undertaken easily without a rest, for example a professional footballer practising advanced dribbling skills.

Massed practice is best for performers with a higher level of skill who want to fine-tune their technique. The skill can become habitual and can be stored in the memory in the form of a motor programme.

One problem with massed practice is that there is no opportunity for input or feedback from the coach during breaks, and the coach is unable to bring the players together during the session to correct faults. Massed practice may also cause fatigue, leading to a dip in performance levels towards the end of the session.

Distributed practice

Distributed practice is when a rest interval is given to allow recuperation. Feedback, coaching and advice on technique can be given during the interval. It is suitable for:

- beginners, who can focus on an early part of a task and may need to rest before moving on to the next part
- performers who are unfit or need to rest
- performers who need encouragement from the coach to improve motivation

It is appropriate for serial skills and complex skills, so that one aspect of the task can be learned before the next part is outlined in the rest interval. For example, a netball coach might give a beginner some basic drills to start with and then offer a rest before the next, more difficult, task is outlined and then attempted. It can also be used to improve safety, since any dangerous elements can be discussed during the break.

Distributed practice is time-consuming but it does ensure that skills are learned thoroughly.

Fixed practice

Fixed practice uses repetition of the same activity to promote over-learning. This ensures that more advanced performers maintain consistency in their performance and that their responses are habitual.

It is appropriate for closed skills that do not require adaptation to the environment, self-paced skills, and simple skills that have a discrete element to them. For example, a national league hockey player might practise penalty flicks or short corners repeatedly so that these skills are performed automatically in a game situation.

Problems of boredom and fatigue can occur if this type of practice is used too much, so it is important for the coach to make sure that the performer is well motivated.

Varied practice

Varied practice involves using different methods to achieve a learning goal, or performing a task in different situations. It aims to provide the performer with the ability to adapt a skill to a range of possible circumstances.

This method is appropriate for open skills, where the sporting environment tends to change. For example, when practising passing techniques in a team game, there will be a variety of drills that suit different situations within the game, such as attacking and defending.

When the skill is externally paced, varied practice may be used because players need to be able to adapt their performance under pressure. For example, when a full court press is used to try to force a mistake by the defensive team in basketball, the attacking team must respond to the added pressure.

Varied practice is often used with beginners, because it allows them to progress when more difficult elements of the task are added to those they are already familiar with. Novice players developing their passing skills may use different drills and small-sided games to help them learn to adapt to the presence of opponents. Varied practice is therefore good for developing experience and may help each player to develop core concepts or schemata for the skill (see pp. 87–89 for more information on schema theory). Variety can also be used to motivate performers.

Varied practice is time-consuming and there can be negative transfer between different tasks.

> ## Tasks to tackle 15.2
>
> Choose a skill from a sport of your choice. Classify the skill and suggest which type of practice you would use to coach it. Give reasons for your choice.

> **Top tip**
>
> Questions on types of practice always require practical examples. Make sure that you can justify your choice of any type of practice by quoting specific examples.

Guidance

Various methods of guidance are used in conjunction with practice to help the performer become familiar with patterns of movement. There are four main methods:

- visual
- verbal
- manual
- mechanical

Visual guidance involves presenting the performer with an accurate picture of the required skill patterns. This may come in the form of a demonstration from the coach, or it could be from a DVD presentation, from a book or from a chart similar to those used by football managers to highlight players' positions and formations.

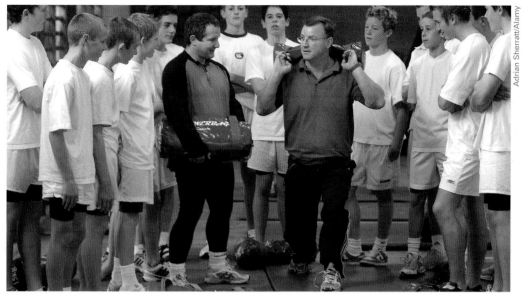

A coach gives visual guidance during a training session

Visual guidance is useful for novices, who may need to see the skill performed before they try to copy it. This gives an initial understanding of the requirements. It can also be used to correct weaknesses in technique, as highlighted by the coach.

When using visual guidance it is important that:

- the demonstration is accurate, so that the performer does not gain a false impression
- the coach does not give too much information as this could cause confusion
- the learner is capable of performing the task accurately

Key terms

Manual guidance: physical support to help a performer in the early stages of learning.
Mechanical guidance: a device used to help a beginner.
Verbal guidance: an explanation of technique.
Visual guidance: a demonstration of technique.

Verbal guidance occurs when the coach gives a full explanation of the coaching points and requirements of the task. The coach should help the performer to gain an understanding of why certain movements are performed.

Verbal guidance can be used for:

- beginners, to help them form a mental picture of the task and to explain the basics of the skill
- for more advanced players, who want to fine-tune their performance
- in team games, to develop tactics and strategies
- giving feedback to a player at the end of the match

Verbal guidance is best used in conjunction with visual guidance. For example, a tennis coach might demonstrate a 'slice' serve and explain that this particular serve is used to move the opponent to the side of the court to pave the way for a winning shot into the empty space.

Verbal guidance should be given in small chunks, because the athlete will be unable to act on a great deal of information given at one time, and in simple language, so that the performer understands all the information given.

Manual and mechanical guidance are physical, hands-on methods used to help the novice performer. Manual guidance involves physical support for the performer. Examples include support for a gymnast doing a handstand, or physically moving the arm of a novice tennis player to achieve the right movement pattern when performing a return shot. Mechanical guidance is the use of a device to support the performer, such as a harness on the trampoline or an armband in swimming. Both these types of guidance can provide early confidence for the learner. He/she will gain an early feel for the skill and be able to accomplish the task with success.

Manual and mechanical guidance can be used in dangerous situations to promote safety. However, these physical types of guidance should be used only in the early stages of learning, otherwise the performer may become dependent on the support and reluctant to perform the skill without it. The performer could also lose motivation if he/she feels unable to undertake the task unaided.

Sports players gain an inner feel for the movement patterns of a task and use an inner sense called kinaesthesis to help them recognise the movements in the muscles. This inner sense can be hindered if too much physical help is offered. Kinaesthesis is discussed in more detail on p. 69.

> **Top tip**
>
> You may be asked for the advantages and disadvantages of certain types of practice or guidance, or about which type of practice or guidance you would use with either a novice or an expert. Remember that if such a question is worth 4 marks, you will score 2 marks for any two advantages and 2 marks for any two disadvantages. In other words, make sure that you answer both parts of the question.

Mental practice

The best improvements in performance are made when physical practice is combined with mental rehearsal. The performer goes over the task in his/her mind, concentrating on the successful aspects of performance. Mental practice should be done in a quiet, calm environment, just before a major event or after a training session with the coach. Figure 15.3 illustrates the relative benefits of physical, mental and combined practice.

Mental rehearsal activates receptors in the muscle spindles, even though no movement takes place, and the athlete gains a sensation of the task. Mental rehearsal improves

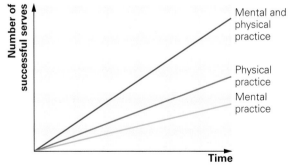

Figure 15.3 Benefits of combined practice

reaction times and confidence. Motivation levels may also increase as the athlete develops a desire to succeed.

Mental practice is becoming popular with sports coaches and players but the technique should be used in different ways for beginners and more experienced athletes. With a beginner the coach could combine mental practice with distributed practice, doing short sessions of mental rehearsal during rest intervals, going over techniques that have just been practised physically. More advanced performers can use quiet times to go over an imminent event in their mind, concentrating on a successful performance. Fine details, strengths to concentrate on and opposition weaknesses may have been highlighted by the coach during training and can be focused on by the performer in preparation for a big match.

Feedback

Feedback is an integral part of information processing, which can help to provide confidence and motivation for the performer. Feedback has a vital role to play in correcting errors and improving performance.

Key term

Feedback: information received to help modify performance.

If you have ever played in a game and felt you had done particularly well, one of the first things you might have done afterwards was to speak to your coach, or your friends who were watching, and ask them how they thought you played. If you watch a performance on television, it is usual for the event to be analysed by a panel of experts, often with the aid of a variety of statistics. The reason that feedback is so popular in sport is that it tends to improve performance. Players who receive feedback perform better than those who don't.

The different types of feedback are shown in Table 15.1.

Table 15.1 Types of feedback

Type	Definition	Phase of learning	Example
Positive	Information about correct technique given to encourage and motivate the player	Cognitive	Praise from the coach to a novice after a good shot
Negative	Information about incorrect technique given to eliminate errors	Associative autonomous	A basketball player being told by a team-mate that a pass was too slow
Intrinsic	Feedback from within the player	Autonomous	A tennis player knowing that she has over-hit a return
Extrinsic	Feedback from an outside source	Cognitive autonomous	Tactical advice from the coach, telling a rugby player not to hold on to the ball for too long before passing
Knowledge of results	Basic information to determine success or failure	Cognitive	A netball player noting that a shot has just missed the goal
Knowledge of performance	More detailed information about technique	Autonomous associative	A netball player being told why the shot missed goal
Concurrent	Feedback given during the performance	Autonomous	The team captain summarising the opponent's strengths at half-time in a game
Terminal	Feedback given after a performance	Cognitive autonomous	The coach summarising the performance after a game

Different types of feedback can occur at the same time. After a game, a coach's summary of a performance could be extrinsic, terminal and negative.

Making feedback effective

Feedback should be given to the performer as soon as possible after the event so that it has maximum impact. It should be target-related and given in language that is understandable and not too technical, especially for beginners. Information given during a game is best broken down into simple chunks. A player will have a lot to think about during the game and will not be able to remember much information.

The coach should be careful to give feedback appropriately. A novice performer will have different needs from those of a more experienced player. Novices need encouragement, so positive feedback should be given to provide motivation. Experienced players can use negative feedback to eliminate errors. A starting point for the beginner could be knowledge of results, and as he/she gains experience, knowledge of performance can be used to fine-tune technique. A beginner who has not yet developed a feel for the game may best use extrinsic feedback as guidelines; more experienced players will realise their own errors using intrinsic feedback.

Practice makes perfect

1 Why is the organisation of a skill important when considering which type of practice to use when teaching that skill? *(2 marks)*

2 What do you understand by the **whole method of practice**? What are the advantages of teaching a skill using the whole method? *(4 marks)*

3 What do you understand by the term **mental rehearsal**? What benefits does mental rehearsal have for the sports performer? *(3 marks)*

AQA AS Physical Education

Answers

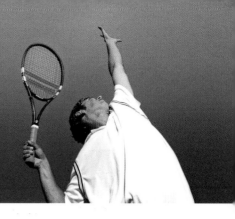

Tasks to tackle

1.1 (page 3)

Smoking, taking drugs, drinking excess alcohol, poor diet, which could lead to obesity, no exercise, late nights

1.2 (page 6)

	Cricketer	Gymnast	Shot-putter	Marathon runner
Stamina	✓			✓
Muscular endurance	✓	✓		✓
Strength	✓	✓	✓	
Speed	✓	✓	✓	
Power	✓	✓	✓	
Flexibility		✓		
Reaction time	✓			
Agility	✓	✓		
Coordination	✓	✓	✓	
Balance		✓	✓	

2.1 (page 11)

Energy requirements without exercise per week	1872 × 7 = 13 104 kcal
Energy requirements including exercise per week	13 104 + 8.5 × 60 × 2 × 5 = 18 204 kcal
% carbohydrates	55–60%
% fats	30–35%
% proteins	5–10%
Suggested meals	Any meal high in carbohydrates and low in fats

3.1 (page 15)

nose → pharynx → larynx → trachea → bronchi → bronchioles → alveoli

4.1 (page 29)

	Before exercise	During exercise	Recovery
Blood pressure changes	Increases	Increases at first; when steady state is reached it decreases	Decreases

5.1 (page 32)

gastrocnemius → vena cava → right atrium → tricuspid valve → right ventricle → semilunar valve → pulmonary artery → lungs → pulmonary vein → left atrium → bicuspid valve → left ventricle → semilunar valve → aorta

6.1 (page 44)

Joint	Joint type	Articulating bones
Ankle	Hinge	Tibia, fibula, talus
Knee	Hinge	Tibia, femur
Hip	Ball and socket	Pelvis, head of femur
Shoulder	Ball and socket	Head of humerus, scapula
Elbow	Hinge	Humerus, radius, ulna

6.2 (page 47)

	Elbow	Shoulder	Hip	Knee	Ankle
Flexion	✓	✓	✓	✓	
Extension	✓	✓	✓	✓	
Abduction		✓	✓		
Adduction		✓	✓		
Rotation		✓	✓		
Horizontal abduction (horizontal flexion)		✓			
Horizontal adduction (horizontal extension)		✓			
Plantarflexion					✓
Dorsiflexion					✓
Circumduction		✓	✓		

6.3 (page 53)

	Movement	Muscle	Type of contraction
1	Flexion	Triceps brachii	Eccentric
2	Extension	Triceps brachii	Concentric
3	—	Triceps brachii	Isometric

6.4 (page 54)

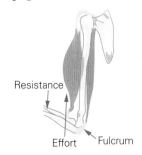

Resistance

Effort   Fulcrum

7.1 (page 61)

Ability	Skill
Innate	Learned
Enduring	Consistent
Foundation of skill	Goal directed

7.2 (page 63)

Any skill may be chosen with associated abilities and fundamental skills, as long as there is a link between them.

7.3 (page 65)

The answers depend on the skill chosen. Refer to the criteria on pp. 63–65 to make sure that your answer is correct.

8.1 (page 70)

The display is the sporting environment from which information is gathered. Selective attention is the process by which information is filtered into relevant and irrelevant items.

8.2 (page 72)

The short-term memory is the working memory. It has a limited capacity, receives information from the sensory stores, and passes and receives information from the long-term memory.

The long-term memory stores motor programmes, has an infinite capacity and lasts for a lifetime. It receives information from the short-term memory and passes this information back to the short-term memory when required.

9.1 (page 80)

Phase of learning	Practice	Feedback	Guidance
Cognitive	Part practice, distributed practice, varied practice	Extrinsic, positive and knowledge of results	Mechanical and manual
Associative	Whole–part–whole, whole, progressive part	Intrinsic and extrinsic using information from the coach, knowledge of performance	Visual and verbal
Autonomous	Whole, fixed, massed	Intrinsic and extrinsic in terms of the coach improving the finer details	Verbal

9.2 (page 84)

Whole approach — the skill should be studied in its entirety, not in parts; so the solution to winning the 1500 m race should not be based just on the last lap.

Problem solving — performance should solve questions that are posed by the situation, such as how you overcome a powerful serve in tennis.

Experience — performers should use what they already know to arrive at the answer, for example how did you combat the serve of a powerful player in your last tennis match?

Understanding — the performer should know the reasons for the answer, for example I will reduce the power of the powerful server by making her move around the court to drain her energy before serving.

9.3 (page 91)

Positive reinforcement is the use of a pleasant stimulus after a correct response to strengthen the S–R bond. Negative reinforcement is the withdrawal of either a pleasant stimulus after an incorrect response or the withdrawal of criticism after a correct response.

10.1 (page 94)

(a) yes, (b) yes, (c) no (you have to do this), (d) no (you have obligations as you are paid to do sport for a living), (e) no (you have to go once you have enrolled)

10.2 (page 96)

(a) Health and fitness; less strain on the NHS; social integration; friendships formed
(b) As (a) plus social control, less crime

10.3 (page 100)

None, as this answer is irrelevant to the question set. The answer links to functions and benefits to society, not to the characteristics. The key to success in exams is to answer the question set.

10.4 (page 101)

Any four from:
- develop physical fitness and skills; improve motor skills in a range of different activities such as games and gymnastics
- develop social skills; improve teamwork in games such as rugby and netball
- prepare for active leisure or a career via enjoyment, skills and qualifications gained during a PE programme (e.g. Community Sports Leadership Award)
- improve quality of life via outdoor and adventurous activities where pupils gain an aesthetic appreciation of the natural environment
- develop cognitive skills — PE involves many activities that require decision making (e.g. tactics) and understanding of rules

10.5 (page 104)

(a) Yes, mountain biking in the natural environment could involve being taught safe techniques of descent (coming down mountains and steep natural hills safely).
(b) No, hockey is normally played on Astroturf, which is artificial.
(c) Yes, as orienteering in the natural environment — being taught how to read a map and take a compass bearing could be part of a pupil's OAA experience.

10.6 (page 105)

Examples: mountain biking, sailing, skiing, orienteering, *if* it is competitive, strict rules are applied (which help determine a winner), there is a national governing body to oversee the activity as a sport, judges or officials are present and extrinsic rewards are available (possibly professional opportunities available).

11.1 (page 107)
Examples should be plentiful and include parks, tennis courts, outdoor basketball courts, skateboard parks, swimming pools, paddling pools, leisure centres and running tracks.

11.2 (page 108)
Key characteristics, two from: run by members or a committee; possibly on a trust or charity basis; financed by members fees and fund raising; aim is to break even or run on profit and loss accounts

Key objectives, two from: grass-roots provision for sport; to increase participation in a certain sport or increase club membership; to provide opportunities to meet up with individuals sharing similar sporting interests; to seek funding to develop their sports club (e.g. from the National Lottery)

12.1 (page 112)
Played regularly during free time; devised initial rules and later standardised rules; allowed inter-house competitions and later inter-school competitions; made structural changes (e.g. time limits, pitch boundaries); role of captain given high status

12.2 (page 113)
Positive use of leisure time to counter bad behaviour; could be played on school grounds, obeying rules developed a positive code of behaviour and fair play; it developed loyalty to the team and teamwork; inter-school fixtures brought the boys together; there was respect for the captain/leader

12.3 (page 116)
For upper/middle classes: captains or leaders in sport and subsequently leaders in society; industrialists, army officers

For the working classes: factory workers; served in the forces — familiarity with weapons important; disciplined, obedient, subservient individuals for workplace and army roles

12.4 (page 118)
Content (1933): more variety, play element introduced, better facilities developed (e.g. gymnasiums), link seen between body and mind

Delivery (1933): introduction to group work, decentralised lessons, teacher began to relate more to the individual, more freedom for teachers

12.5 (page 119)
Content: free movement, dance/educational gymnastics, creativity, apparatus-based, active/energetic

Teaching style: guidance/discovery style/problem solving, teacher–pupil interaction, group work, teachers devised their own work

12.6 (page 129)

Increase links between the two, school–club links, share coaches and facilities; observe government policy (e.g. PESSCL, sports colleges, SSCos); offer discounts and subsidised use of facilities; put on taster days; offer different ways of participating (e.g. recreational or competitive); increase awareness of health and fitness issues

12.7 (page 132)

Any three from: Active Schools, Active Communities, Active Sports, Get Active; sports colleges, SSCos; Activemark, Sportsmark, Sports Partnership Mark; PESSCL; National Junior Sport Programme, TOPs; Sport Action Zones

12.8 (page 134)

Run by Youth Sport Trust, for 7–11 year olds, part of Sport England's Active Schools project; in partnership with LEAs, SSCos, NGBs; supports National Curriculum PE; provides sport-specific, age-related equipment in a range of activities; provides illustrated resource cards for teaching skills and setting up modified games; provides training for teachers by qualified trainers

12.9 (page 136)

It can be played at any age; it is a good physical activity with health benefits; it has a handicap system of play, which means that all abilities, ages and genders can play or compete together; it is a sociable game; it can be played recreationally for social benefits

13.1 (page 140)

Examples might include: lack of free time (due to academic work commitments), lack of money, norms and stereotypes of society against participation in certain activities (e.g. rugby if you are female, dance if you are male), lack of clubs, poor PE experiences put you off participation

13.2 (page 143)

Stereotypes and old-fashioned attitudes; verbal or sexual harassment; few clubs, restrictive membership clauses and fewer competitions; lower funding, costs too high; less media coverage, fewer role models

13.3 (page 146)

Yes: some sports require higher social status to participate (e.g. polo); some sports have strong working-class links (e.g. darts, rugby league)

No: social class is less well defined today than in the past; participation is now considered a right for all; sports show a greater mixing of social classes than before (e.g. rugby union, horse-riding)

15.1 (page 165)

Task	Performer
Danger	Motivation
Open or closed skill	Ability
Organisation	Age
Complexity	Experience

15.2 (page 170)

The answer depends on the skill chosen. Refer to the text to ensure that the answer is correct.

Practice makes perfect

Chapter 1 (page 6)

1   Any two of the following for 2 marks: power, speed, stamina (or equivalent), flexibility, coordination, muscular endurance, strength, balance; 1 mark for a correct example of one of these.

2   Any two for 2 marks: amount of work done or effort; per unit of time; speed × strength

3   Any two for 2 marks: speed, strength, flexibility, agility

4   Fitness: the ability to perform daily tasks without undue fatigue. *(1 mark)*
Health: a state of complete physical, mental, and social well-being. *(1 mark)*

Chapter 2 (page 12)

1   Iron: haemoglobin/red blood cells *(1 mark)*; enhances the transport of oxygen *(1 mark)*; improved stamina *(1 mark)*
Calcium: bones *(1 mark)*; important for nerve transmission and muscle contraction *(1 mark)*
(max. 3 marks)

2   A marathon runner requires: more carbohydrate *(1 mark)*; for energy *(1 mark).*
A weightlifter requires: more protein *(1 mark)*; for muscle growth *(1 mark).*
(max. 3 marks)

3   Carbohydrate is the main energy fuel for both aerobic and anaerobic work. *(1 mark)*
Fats are the secondary energy fuel for low-intensity work. *(1 mark)*
Proteins are for tissue growth and repair. *(1 mark)*

Chapter 3 (page 22)

1   Any four for 4 marks:
   - increase in carbon dioxide/decrease in pH of the blood
   - detected by chemoreceptors

- nerve impulses sent to the medulla/respiratory centre
- phrenic/intercostal nerves
- deeper and faster breathing

2   Arterio-venous difference is the difference between the oxygen content of arterial and that of venous blood. *(1 mark)*
    It increases during exercise because the muscles use more oxygen. *(1 mark)*

3   Any three for 3 marks:
    - increase in blood temperature
    - increase in blood carbon dioxide
    - increase in the acidity of blood
    - Bohr shift

    Any one for 1 mark:
    - less saturation of haemoglobin with oxygen as a result
    - therefore an increase in oxygen release

4   Tidal volume is the amount of air breathed in *or* out per breath. *(1 mark)*
    It increases during exercise. *(1 mark)*

5   Any four for 4 marks:
    - gas flows from an area of high pressure to low pressure
    - (partial) pressure/concentration of oxygen is high in the lungs/alveoli and low in the blood
    - therefore oxygen diffuses down the diffusion gradient into the blood
    - 3% dissolves in the plasma
    - 97% combines with haemoglobin

6   Any three for 3 marks:
    - the diaphragm contracts, increasing the volume of the thoracic cavity
    - the external intercostals muscles contract, pulling the ribs upwards and outwards, increasing the volume of the thoracic cavity
    - this has the net effect of lowering the pressure and air moves into the lungs
    - expiration is passive

Chapter 4 (page 30)

1   Any three for 3 marks:
    - skeletal muscle pump — muscles change shape when they contract and relax, and this squeezes the veins, pushing blood through
    - respiratory pump — changes in thoracic pressure cause a squeezing effect on the veins
    - valves prevent backflow
    - smooth muscle in the veins help squeeze blood back towards the heart

2 Brain function/activity needs to be maintained both during exercise and at rest. *(1 mark)*

The brain needs glucose/oxygen. *(1 mark)*

3 Any three for 3 marks:
- active muscles require oxygen
- during exercise, less blood flows to the gut
- if there is food in the gut, blood will be redirected for digestion
- this reduces the blood to the working muscles
- which will reduce performance
- the performer may feel sick

4 Any two for 2 marks: combines with haemoglobin; dissolves in plasma; as bicarbonate/hydrogen carbonate

5 Any three for 3 marks:
- increase in carbon dioxide/drop in pH
- detected by chemoreceptors
- impulse sent to the medulla/vasomotor centre
- vasoconstriction in arterioles to non-essential organs
- vasodilation in arterioles to working muscles
- precapillary sphincters control blood flow/open leading to muscles/closed leading to non-essential organs

6 120/80 *(1 mark)*; blood pressure/systolic pressure increases *(1 mark)*

Chapter 5 (page 40)

1 Any three for 3 marks:
- detected by chemoreceptors
- nerve impulse sent to medulla/cardiac control centre
- impulse sent via sympathetic system/cardiac accelerator nerve
- to SA node/SAN

2 Any three for 3 marks:
- hypertrophy of the cardiac muscle
- athlete's heart
- bradycardia
- increase in resting stroke volume
- increase in ejection fraction
- increase in maximum cardiac output
- increased capillarisation of the heart muscle

3 Heart rate increases/anticipatory rise *(1 mark)*; due to the effects of adrenaline *(1 mark)*.

Answers

4   Bradycardia is a reduction in **resting** heart rate/below 60 bpm. *(1 mark)*
     Athlete's heart is an increase in chamber size. *(1 mark)*

5   Cardiac output is the amount of blood leaving the left ventricle per minute. *(1 mark)*
     Stroke volume is the amount of blood leaving the left ventricle per beat. *(1 mark)*
     Relationship: cardiac output = stroke volume × heart rate *(1 mark)*

6   Stroke volume increases *(1 mark)*; cardiac output does not change *(1 mark)*

Chapter 6 (page 58)
1   **(a)** Drive

Joint	Movement	Agonist	Antagonist	Plane	Axis	Type of contraction	Lever system
Hip	Extension	Gluteus maximus	Iliopsoas	Sagittal	Transverse	Concentric	Third
Knee	Extension	Quadriceps	Hamstrings	Sagittal	Transverse	Concentric	Third
Ankle	Plantarflexion	Gastrocnemius	Tibialis anterior	Sagittal	Transverse	Concentric	Second

(b) Recovery

Joint	Movement	Agonist	Antagonist	Plane	Axis	Type of contraction	Lever system
Hip	Flexion	Hip flexors (iliopsoas)	Gluteus maximus	Sagittal	Transverse	Concentric	Third
Knee	Flexion	Hamstrings	Quadriceps	Sagittal	Transverse	Concentric	Third
Ankle	Dorsiflexion	Tibialis anterior	Gastrocnemius	Sagittal	Transverse	Concentric	Second

2   Second order *(1 mark)*

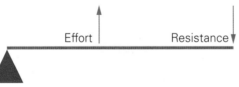

Effort   Resistance

Fulcrum

Correct labels *(1 mark)* in correct order *(1 mark)*

3   Mechanical advantage (any two for 2 marks):
     - large effort arm and shorter resistance arm
     - heavy loads can be moved but only over a short distance
     - does not need a lot of force

     Mechanical disadvantage (any two for 2 marks):
     - large resistance arm and shorter effort arm
     - cannot move as heavy a load
     - but can move it faster

AQA AS Physical Education

Chapter 7 (page 66)

1 There is no general ability in sport because abilities are specific to the task and occur in small groups. For example, coordination and power are the abilities underpinning the tennis serve.

2 A continuum shows the range along which a skill matches certain criteria and the extent to which the skill matches those criteria. For example, in tennis a return of serve is classified as an open skill because it is affected by the environment. A football pass is also open but because it involves more decision-making it is more open than the return of serve in tennis. A continuum also shows how skills can change with the situation. For example, a basketball pass is open in a game but closed in practice.

Chapter 8 (page 77)

1 Any four for four marks:
- Use mental rehearsal to go over the performance in the mind.
- Use different types of practice to ensure the drills are stored in the memory.
- Point out similarities with information already stored, for example between a known tennis serve and an overarm volleyball serve.
- Use praise and reinforcement.
- Break the information into chunks, and make it relevant and meaningful to the performer.

2 Reaction time is the time from the onset of the stimulus to the onset of the response. *(1 mark)*
Movement time is the time from the start of the task to its completion. *(1 mark)*
Response time is the time from the onset of the stimulus to the completion of the task. *(1 mark)*
In a 100 m sprint, reaction time is the time from hearing the gun to leaving the blocks, movement time is the time from leaving the blocks to hitting the finish line, and response time is the time from hearing the gun to hitting the finish line. Response time is reaction time plus movement time.

Chapter 9 (page 92)

1 The coach could offer praise, reinforcement, rewards *(1 mark)*; use Thorndike's law of effect to give a satisfier after a correct response or an annoyer after an incorrect response *(1 mark)*; use the law of exercise, which states that practice is needed *(1 mark)*; set tasks that the performer is capable of completing successfully (the law of readiness) *(1 mark)*

2
- Positive transfer occurs when the learning and performance of one skill is aided by the learning and performance of another *(1 mark)*. When two skills have a similar shape, for example a tennis serve and an overarm volleyball serve, positive transfer might occur when knowledge of one is used to help the other *(1 mark)*.

- Negative transfer is when one skill hinders the learning and performance of another *(1 mark)*. The skills may have some similarity. For example, a tennis serve and a badminton serve are both used in court games, but the actions are different and therefore confusion between the two causes negative transfer *(1 mark)*.
- Zero transfer occurs when there is no impact on the learning and performance of one skill from another. *(1 mark)* For example, rock climbing and swimming produce neither positive nor negative effects. *(1 mark)*
- Bilateral transfer is when a skill is transferred across the body from one limb to another. *(1 mark)* A right-footed football player using his/her left foot to shoot and pass is an example. *(1 mark)*
- Retroactive transfer occurs when a current skill is taken back to one already learned. *(1 mark)* Someone who plays badminton through the winter and goes back to play tennis in summer may find that his/her serve is affected by transfer. *(1 mark)*
- Proactive transfer is when a learned skill is used to develop a skill currently being practised. *(1 mark)* A netball player might use the netball pass she knows to help learn a basketball pass she is trying to develop. *(1 mark)*

Chapter 10 (page 105)

1   Any four for 4 marks:
- competitive/serious
- structured/strict rules/time limit/space boundaries
- rules externally enforced/officials present
- extrinsic rewards available
- involves commitment/endeavour/dedication
- tactical/strategic
- high levels of physical skill/prowess
- sportsmanship

2   Physical activity in the natural environment *(1 mark)* in a person's free time *(1 mark)* with individuals having a choice *(1 mark)* of how to spend that time.

3   Active leisure is free time spent in a physically energetic way, e.g. physical recreation. *(max. 1 mark)*
Purposes of active leisure (for individuals and society) *(max. 3 marks)*:
- increase physical fitness/mental health
- social control/decrease crime
- increase self-esteem
- increase social integration
- create employment opportunities/economic benefits
- friendships formed

4   Any four for 4 marks:
- increases health and fitness

- develops social skills
- develops emotional/moral skills
- improves cognitive skills/decision making
- develops imagination/creativity
- fun/enjoyment

5 Any three for 3 marks:
- appreciation of the natural environment
- conservation awareness
- development of survival skills/assessment of risk
- development of cognitive skills/decision making
- development of leadership skills/teamwork/trust
- preparation for active leisure/a career

Chapter 11 (page 109)

1 Public sector, private sector, voluntary sector *(3 marks)*

2 Private sector: profit making/exclusive *(1 mark)*
Public sector: social needs met/equal opportunities important *(1 mark)*
Voluntary sector: development of interest in a particular sport/increasing membership of a sports club *(1 mark)*

3 Local authority/local government: provides a service for the local community; via a range of activities; needs to give value for money from council tax/'Best Value'; needs to break even/cover running costs *(max. 2 marks)*
Private sector: profit-orientated; services aimed at a socially narrower range of customers/exclusivity; high-quality facilities/equipment/services *(max. 2 marks)*

Chapter 12 (page 137)

1 Any two for 2 marks:
- increase health and fitness of working classes
- increase familiarity with weapons
- increase obedience/discipline

2 Any three for 3 marks:
- became more child-centred
- children's need were taken into account (e.g. physical/social/emotional needs)
- increased educational focus/seen as individuals
- decision making/creativity encouraged
- more emphasis on fun/enjoyment

3 Any two for 2 marks: role as coach, official, choreographer, spectator, captain/leader, critical performer; observation and analysis

4   Any three for 3 marks:

- 2 hours is only a guideline/not compulsory, so if the head teacher of the school views PE as a low-status subject, it might not get 2 hours on the timetable, particularly at Key Stage 4
- PE has lower status than other subjects (e.g. maths) and is considered less important than more 'academic' subjects
- timetable restrictions (e.g. exam demands at Key Stage 4)
- lack of specialist PE teachers
- lack of finance/budget restriction affects facilities/equipment/activities experienced, e.g. OAA are relatively expensive and may not be experienced in National Curriculum PE by large numbers of pupils as a result

5   Any four for 4 marks:

- develop specific initiatives/policies to increase participation in target groups
- arrange funding for target groups/fund mass participation initiatives
- employ sport development officers to promote sport in target groups
- invest in facility provision, to make the sport more accessible and affordable
- run campaigns to dispel myths that might deter certain groups from participating
- provide positive role models to follow (e.g. via media coverage)
- positive discrimination in terms of target groups when employing officials in NGBs

Chapter 13 (page 146)

1   Any two for 2 marks:

- a lot of people taking part in sporting activities
- grass-roots/foundation stage of the sports development pyramid
- requires discrimination to be eliminated
- suggests social policy/government agency involvement to ensure this

2   Any four for 4 marks:

- equal opportunities/war effort/Sex Discrimination Act
- more media coverage/role models
- encouragement via school PE programmes/extra-curricular opportunities
- FA more approving/more clubs offering competitive opportunities
- reduced stereotypes/more socially acceptable
- more leisure time/disposable income available to women

3   Any five for 5 marks:

- social status/working classes least likely to participate
- family/peers influence
- religion/culture/race issues
- amount of leisure time available

- gender
- age
- disability
- discrimination
- media coverage/role models
- access to facilities/clubs/coaches/amount of disposable income
- PE experience

Chapter 14 (page 163)

1   Sit-and-reach test. Any two for 2 marks:
- performer adopts a sitting position against a box
- he/she reaches forward as far as possible and holds
- distance stretched is recorded

2   Any two for 2 marks:
- oxidises and removes lactic acid
- maintains the skeletal muscle pump
- reduces blood pooling in the veins
- keeps heart rate elevated

3   Any two for 2 marks:
- can be adapted to suit most types of performer
- can work any of the three energy systems
- can be made more sport specific

Chapter 15 (page 174)

1   Organisation of a skill refers to the degree to which that skill can be broken down. If the skill can be broken down — such as the clearly defined arm action and leg action in a swimming stroke — it can be taught in parts *(1 mark)*. If the skill is hard to break down — such as the quick action of a golf swing — whole practice must be used *(1 mark)*.

2   Whole practice is when the skill is taught in its entirety, with the subroutines intact *(1 mark)*. It promotes fluency and understanding and may help to develop motor programmes *(1 mark)*. The skill is learned with efficiency *(1 mark)* and the link between the stimulus and the response can be developed *(1 mark)*.

3   Mental rehearsal is the process of going through the skill in the mind *(1 mark)*. It helps to store images in the memory *(1 mark)*, builds motor programmes *(1 mark)* and improves reaction time *(1 mark)*. Mental rehearsal allows practice to take place even when the performer is injured *(1 mark)*. There is evidence to suggest that a combination of mental and physical practice improves performance. *(max. 3 marks)*

Index

Index

AQA AS Physical Education

Index

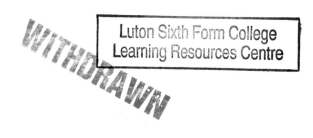